Code Blue:
Cardiac Arrest
and
Resuscitation

MICKEY S. EISENBERG, M.D., Ph.D.

Professor, Department of Medicine
University of Washington
Director, Emergency Medicine Service
University Hospital
Medical Advisor, Emergency Medical Services Division
Co-Director, Center for Evaluation of Emergency Medical Services
King County Health Department
Seattle, Washington

RICHARD O. CUMMINS, M.D., M.P.H., M.Sc.

Professor, Department of Medicine
University of Washington
Attending Physician, Emergency Medicine Service
University Hospital
Director, EMT-Defibrillation Program
Emergency Medical Services Division
Co-Director, Center for Evaluation of Emergency Medical Services
King County Health Department
Seattle, Washington

MARY T. HO, M.D., M.P.H.

Acting Assistant Professor, Department of Medicine
University of Washington
Attending Physician, Emergency Medicine Service
University Hospital
Medical Advisor, Emergency Medical Services Division
Co-Director, Center for Evaluation of Emergency Medical Services
King County Health Department
Seattle, Washington

W.B. SAUNDERS COMPANY
Harcourt Brace Jovanovich, Inc.

Philadelphia   London   Toronto
Montreal   Sydney   Tokyo

Blue Books Series is a trademark of the W.B. Saunders Company

W. B. SAUNDERS COMPANY
Harcourt Brace Jovanovich, Inc.

The Curtis Center
Independence Square West
Philadelphia, PA 19106

Library of Congress Cataloging-in-Publication Data

Eisenberg, Mickey S.

Code blue.

(Blue book series)

1. Cardiac arrest.   2. Cardiac resuscitation.
   I. Cummins, Richard O.   II. Ho, Mary T.
   III. Title. [DNLM: 1. Heart Arrest.
   2. Resuscitation.   WG 205 E36c]

RC685.C173E37   1987   616.1′29   87–12816

ISBN 0–7216–1822–7

Editor: John Dyson
Designer: Terri Siegel
Production Manager: Pete Faber
Manuscript Editor: Erika Shapiro
Cover Designer: Sharon Iwanczuk
Illustration Coordinator: Walt Verbitski
Indexer: Erika Shapiro

Code Blue: Cardiac Arrest and Resuscitation   ISBN   0–7216–1822–7

Last digit is the print number: 9   8   7   6   5   4   3   2

INTRODUCTORY NOTE

Each volume in the Saunders Blue Books™ Series is intended to be a practical aid for primary care physicians, house officers, and medical students in clinical training. Each Blue Book presents the latest diagnostic and therapeutic information pertinent to its clinical field. Above all else, these books are intended to be useful in the real world of providing daily patient care. Their convenient format allows maximal retrieval of relevant information in a minimum of time.

Our Series derives its name from the "Blue Series"—the first books published by the W. B. Saunders Company almost 100 years ago. That Series, like its modern descendant, was intended to sort out important scientific and clinical facts that would aid the physician or the student in training. Today, as medical information grows exponentially, health professionals recognize their obligation both to remain current and to select from the engulfing sea of clinical data those particular pieces that will aid them in their practice. The volumes in Saunders Blue Books™ Series will help them achieve these goals. They should be regarded as portable clinical tools—useful, always on call, and ready to help when needed.

MICKEY S. EISENBERG, M.D., PH.D.
Consulting Editor

CONTRIBUTORS

Editors

MICKEY S. EISENBERG, M.D., Ph.D.
Associate Professor, Department of Medicine, University of Washington; Director, Emergency Medicine Service, University Hospital; Medical Advisor, Emergency Medical Services Division, and Co-Director, Center for Evaluation of Emergency Medical Services, King County Health Department, Seattle, WA
(The Patient; Arrhythmias; Near-Drowning; Legal Considerations; Documentation)

RICHARD O. CUMMINS, M.D., M.P.H., M.Sc.
Associate Professor, Department of Medicine, University of Washington; Attending Physician, Emergency Medicine Service, University Hospital; Director, EMT-Defibrillation Program, Emergency Medical Services Division, and Co-Director, Center for Evaluation of Emergency Medical Services, King County Health Department, Seattle, WA
(Adult Basic Cardiopulmonary Resuscitation; Airway Management; Defibrillation; Emergency Cardiac Pacing)

MARY T. HO, M.D.
Acting Assistant Professor, Department of Medicine, University of Washington; Attending Physician, Emergency Medicine Service, University Hospital; Medical Advisor, Emergency Medical Services Division, and Co-Director, Center for Evaluation of Emergency Medical Services, King County Health Department, Seattle, WA
(Airway Management; Central Venous Lines; Additional Techniques; Drugs Used in Resuscitation; Traumatic Cardiac Arrest; Post-Resuscitation Care)

Contributing Authors

NORMAN S. ABRAMSON, M.D.
Assistant Professor of Critical Care Medicine, Associate Director for Clinical Affairs, Resuscitation Research Center, University of Pittsburgh, Pittsburgh, PA
(Cerebral Resuscitation)

FREDERICK M. BURKLE, JR., M.D., M.P.H., F.A.A.P., F.A.C.E.P.
Medical Staff Director, Maui Memorial Hospital, Wailuku, Maui, HA; Formerly Residency Director, Department of Emergency

Medicine, Madigan Army Medical Center, Tacoma, WA
(Code Organization)

CHARLES GUILDNER, M.D.
Anesthesia Associates, Everett, WA
(Adult Basic Cardiopulmonary Resuscitation)

THOMAS HEARNE, Ph.D.
Program Analyst, Emergency Medical Services Division, King
County Health Department, Seattle, WA
(Introduction)

KAREN KILIAN, R.N., B.S.N., C.C.R.N.
Flight Nurse, Airlift Northwest, Seattle, WA
(Pediatric Cardiac Arrest)

RITA S. McCLARTY, R.N.C.
Outreach Coordinator, Children's Orthopedic Hospital and Medi-
cal Center, Seattle, WA
(Pediatric Cardiac Arrest)

JOSEPH ORNATO, M.D.
Associate Professor of Medicine, Section of Emergency Medical
Services, Medical College of Virginia, Virginia Commonwealth
University, Richmond, VA
(Near-Drowning; Hypothermia)

MATHEW M. RICE, M.D.
Residency Director, Department of Emergency Medicine, Madigan
Army Medical Center, Tacoma, WA
(Code Organization)

PETER SAFAR, M.D.
Distinguished Service Professor of Resuscitation Medicine and
Director, Resuscitation Research Center, University of Pittsburgh,
Pittsburgh, PA
(Cerebral Resuscitation)

ARTHUR SAUNDERS, M.D.
Associate Professor, Section of Emergency Medicine, Department
of Surgery, University of Arizona Health Sciences Center, Tucson,
AZ
(Acid-Base Balance)

STANLEY J. STAMM, M.D.
Clinical Professor of Pediatrics, University of Washington; Head,
Cardiology Division, Children's Orthopedic Hospital and Medical
Center, Seattle, WA
(Pediatric Cardiac Arrest)

PREFACE

There is nothing more dramatic or challenging in medicine than the management of cardiac arrest. Suddenly, lying before the doctor, nurse, or paramedic is the moment of truth. There is no time to prepare. There is no leisurely opportunity to read a textbook. There is no chance for consultation. The awful jaws of death gape open, about to close forever, and only knowledge and skill can afford a chance to snatch life back.

If handled properly, a resuscitation attempt, regardless of the outcome, can afford one the satisfaction (never the complacency) of having acted responsibly and professionally, of having brought to the patient the best that medical science has to offer. Such a feeling can help blunt the awesome and terrible emotions of having confronted death. A poorly handled resuscitation attempt, on the other hand, can give one the unpleasant feeling of having failed as a professional, with the hope that such a bad experience will at least result in motivation to be better prepared the next time.

The ability to manage a cardiac arrest is a skill every physician, critical care nurse, and paramedic should have. Unfortunately, cardiac arrests cannot be scheduled like office visits. A physician or other health professional is likely to be thrust into the role of managing a cardiac arrest at any time and at any place. The public expects a health professional, by virtue of his or her training, to know what to do in this most critical moment.

The purpose of this book is to prepare and provide. The material can prepare a physician, nurse, and paramedic with the necessary knowledge and skills, and, by virtue of its format, can provide instant information and guidance in the management of cardiac arrest. The book is not a textbook and DOES NOT replace the training or information provided by the American Heart Association's Advanced Cardiac Life Support course. We wish every health professional could take this course and be familiar with the contents of the *Textbook of Advanced Cardiac Life Support* (American Heart Association). The contents of the *Textbook of Advanced Cardiac Life Support* are based upon the *Standards and Guidelines for Emergency Cardiac Care* issued by the American Heart Association and published as a special supplement in the *Journal of the American Medical Association* (JAMA). The standards and guidelines are revised approximately every 5 years; they were last updated in July 1985, and were subsequently published in JAMA in June 1986 (Vol. 255, pp. 2905–2985).

This book supplements and complements the material in the most recent edition of the *Textbook of Advanced Cardiac Life*

Support, as well as the 1986 *Standards and Guidelines for Emergency Cardiac Care*. The information is intended to be clinically relevant. Thus, major emphasis is placed on specific and detailed therapy. There is little discussion of pathophysiology. All therapeutic information is presented in a readily accessible format. The book is intended to be on hand when needed.

We have done our best to provide state-of-the-art information on the management of cardiac arrest. We have also tried to identify where controversy exists.

As clinicians and researchers involved in cardiac arrest and resuscitation, we know that skill and knowledge make a difference. We also know that not everyone in cardiac arrest can be or should be resuscitated. There is a time for life and a time for death. There is also a time to be prepared.

MICKEY S. EISENBERG
RICHARD O. CUMMINS
MARY T. HO

ACKNOWLEDGMENTS

The editors wish to thank Dr. Nicholas J. Juele for suggesting the idea of a clinical manual on cardiac arrest and resuscitation. It has been a pleasure to work with the editors and production staff of the W. B. Saunders Company. We particularly appreciate the constant support of John Dyson, medical editor. Thanks also to Judy Prentice for her tireless typing and patience with the word processor (despite a crash or two).

CONTENTS

INTRODUCTION
CARDIAC ARREST AND RESUSCITATION IN A
   HISTORICAL CONTEXT 1

1
THE PATIENT IN SUDDEN CARDIAC ARREST............. 7

EPIDEMIOLOGY.. 7
RHYTHM 7
ETIOLOGY 8
RISK FACTORS 8
PATHOPHYSIOLOGY 9
DETERMINANTS OF SURVIVAL 10
FATE FACTORS... 11
PROGRAM FACTORS.. 12
TIERED RESPONSE SYSTEM 14
CARDIAC ARREST IN THE HOSPITAL...................... 14
TYPES OF CARDIAC ARREST............................. 15
SPECTRUM OF ARREST..................................... 17
ANTICIPATING AND PREVENTING CARDIAC ARREST..... 18
OUTCOMES FOLLOWING CARDIAC ARREST 19
MEASURES OF MORBIDITY 23

2
CODE ORGANIZATION 26

PHASES IN CODE ORGANIZATION......................... 26
   Anticipation... 26
   Entry 28
   Resuscitation 28
   Maintenance.. 30
   Family Notification 30
   Transfer 31
   Critique.. 31

3
ADULT BASIC CARDIOPULMONARY RESUSCITATION ... 32

MAJOR FEATURES OF BASIC CPR: THE ABCs 32
   Airway... 32
   Breathing 34
   Circulation 36

TWO-PERSON CPR.. 38
    Airway Management During Basic CPR.................... 39
    The Obstructed Airway...................................... 40
    Open-Chest Cardiac Massage 43

4

AIRWAY MANAGEMENT 45

DEVICES USED IN BASIC LIFE SUPPORT 47
DEVICES USED IN ADVANCED LIFE SUPPORT............ 51
    Endotracheal Intubation..................................... 53
    Transtracheal Catheter Insufflation......................... 55
    Cricothyrotomy.. 56
MECHANICAL VENTILATION................................. 57

5

CENTRAL VENOUS LINES.................................... 61

INTERNAL JUGULAR CANNULATION....................... 61
SUBCLAVIAN VEIN CANNULATION......................... 63
FEMORAL VEIN CANNULATION 65
VENOUS CUTDOWN... 67

6

DEFIBRILLATION 70

PHYSIOLOGY 71
DEFIBRILLATORS.. 74
TECHNIQUE.. 77
TROUBLESHOOTING 78
SPECIAL TOPICS AND FUTURE DIRECTION............... 80

7

ADDITIONAL TECHNIQUES.................................. 86

PERICARDIOCENTESIS....................................... 86
INTRACARDIAC INJECTION 87

8

**EMERGENCY CARDIAC PACING: TRANCUTANEOUS
PACING, TRANSVENOUS PACING, AND
TRANSTHORACIC PACING.**.............................. 90

TRANCUTANEOUS PACEMAKERS 90
TRANSVENOUS PACEMAKERS 100
TRANSTHORACIC PACEMAKERS 101

9

DRUGS USED IN RESUSCITATION...................... 103

ANTIARRHYTHMICS 103
  Lidocaine 103
  Procainamide... 103
  Bretylium 104
  Atropine 104
  Verapamil.. 105
  Propranolol 105
ADRENERGIC AGONISTS.............................. 106
  Isoproterenol... 106
  Epinephrine... 106
  Norepinephrine 107
  Dopamine 107
  Dobutamine... 108
VASODILATING AGENTS 108
  Nitroglycerin 108
  Nitroprusside 110
  Nifedipine... 110
  Diuretics.. 111
  Furosemide and Ethacrynic Acid 111
MISCELLANEOUS AGENTS............................. 111
  Digoxin 111
  Morphine 112
  Calcium... 112
  Sodium Bicarbonate 112
  Amrinone 113

10

ARRHYTHMIAS 114

MANAGEMENT... 114
  Guidelines and Protocols 114
VENTRICULAR FIBRILLATION 115
VENTRICULAR FLUTTER 120
VENTRICULAR TACHYCARDIA 121
ASYSTOLE 123
ELECTROMECHANICAL DISSOCIATION.................. 125
IDIOVENTRICULAR RHYTHM 127
PAROXYSMAL SUPRAVENTRICULAR TACHYCARDIA 127
ATRIAL FLUTTER 130
ATRIAL FIBRILLATION 131
BRADYCARDIA AND AV BLOCK.......................... 134
PREMATURE VENTRICULAR CONTRACTIONS 137

11

ACID-BASE BALANCE................................... 142

IMPORTANCE OF VENTILATION.......................... 142
ARTERIAL-VENOUS CO_2 GAP 142
ARTERIAL BLOOD GASES................................ 144
BICARBONATE THERAPY CONTROVERSY 145
CLINICAL RECOMMENDATIONS.......................... 148

12

CEREBRAL RESUSCITATION 149

PATHOPHYSIOLOGY 150
THERAPEUTIC APPROACH................................ 153
    Brain-Specific Therapies 159

13

PEDIATRIC CARDIAC ARREST........................... 163

CAUSES OF RESPIRATORY ARREST IN CHILDREN...... 163
CAUSES OF CARDIAC ARREST IN CHILDREN............ 165
BASIC LIFE SUPPORT.................................... 166
ADVANCED LIFE SUPPORT 168
INTRAVENOUS ACCESS................................... 173
EMERGENCY MEDICATIONS 179

14

TRAUMATIC CARDIAC ARREST 183

GENERAL CONSIDERATIONS 183
INITIAL THERAPY.. 183
    Emergency Thoracotomy 183
    MAST 186
OUTCOME 191

15

NEAR-DROWNING 192

DEFINITIONS.. 192
INCIDENCE.. 192
CLINICAL PRESENTATION................................ 192
INITIAL TREATMENT (Prehospital) 193
PREHOSPITAL ADVANCED LIFE SUPPORT
    PROCEDURES... 194
EMERGENCY DEPARTMENT PROCEDURES.............. 194
PROGNOSIS 195

16
HYPOTHERMIA 196

DEFINITION AND ETIOLOGY 196
CLINICAL FEATURES 196
TREATMENT 197

17
LEGAL CONSIDERATIONS 201

LEGAL QUESTIONS IN CRITICAL CARE 201

18
POST-RESUSCITATION CARE 208

STEPS IN POST-RESUSCITATION MANAGEMENT 208
MANAGEMENT IN THE INTENSIVE CARE UNIT 209

19
DOCUMENTATION 211

APPENDICES 213

I. TABLE OF ACLS DRUGS 214
II. POCKET SUMMARY OF ACLS DRUGS 225
III. ABBREVIATED ACLS PROTOCOLS 227

INDEX 231

INTRODUCTION

CARDIAC ARREST AND RESUSCITATION IN A HISTORICAL CONTEXT

This book discusses the latest therapies in the management of cardiac arrest. Yet it is also true that "there is nothing new under the sun." The three major elements of modern resuscitation—namely ventilation, chest compression, and defibrillation—have a history dating back centuries. Unfortunately, each history was a separate history, with false starts and dead ends. It was not until the early 1960s that the three came together, resulting in modern resuscitation, which has evolved rapidly since.

EARLY HISTORY

Biblical and Talmudic texts, as well as scripts from ancient near-eastern civilizations, contain some of the earliest accounts of resuscitation. These attempts, embedded in religious beliefs and attitudes, attributed successful resuscitation to divine intervention. One of the most famous of these is the biblical account of the Hebrew prophet Elisha's successful resuscitation of a child, in which mouth-to-mouth respiration was used (2 Kings:3–5). Beginning in the seventeenth century, experimental and scientific methods were used to establish the physiologic basis for cardiac resuscitation. The discovery of the circulation of blood was described by William Harvey in 1628. In a series of extensive experiments, Harvey showed the relationship between heartbeat and blood circulation, and discovered the link between the circulatory and respiratory systems.

VENTILATION

The first scientifically documented case of successful mouth-to-mouth resuscitation was presented to the Royal Society of London in 1745 by William Tossach, a Scottish surgeon. He successfully resuscitated a miner, who had collapsed from smoke inhalation, by administering mouth-to-mouth respiration followed by the conventional techniques of bleeding and smelling salts.

Many techniques of ventilation have been proposed. Between 1890 and 1950, more than 100 manual techniques for providing artificial ventilation were put forth. Each technique attempted to provide adequate ventilation to unconscious patients by alternatively producing and releasing pressure on the chest or abdomen, thus causing expiration and inspiration. The means by which pressure was produced on the patient's chest varied. Early artificial techniques employed means such as wrapping the patient's chest with a narrow fabric strip (Dalrymple method, 1831), rolling the patient from side to side (Marshall Hall method, 1856), and pressing the patient's arms against his chest (Silvester method, 1858). In 1902, E. A. Shafer proposed a new method, which utilized compressions on the lower back of the patient. In 1932, this technique was modified by Holger Nielsen, a colonel in the Danish Army, to back pressure–arm lift. The latter two techniques, with modifications, were popular and widely used into the 1950s.

CHEST COMPRESSIONS

In 1796, chest compression similar to that used today was described by Danish physicians Herholdt and Rafn. They noted that their technique was useful for inducing artificial respiration and was clearly preferable to mouth-to-mouth ventilation, which they deplored as ". . . toilsome and lothsome."

Direct cardiac massage methods were first attempted in humans in 1880, during an unsuccessful effort to resuscitate a patient who died during goiter surgery. By 1903, seven attempts had been made to resuscitate patients by direct cardiac massage: the first success was accomplished by the Norwegian surgeon Igelsrud in 1901. In 1904, the American surgeon Crile successfully resuscitated a patient using a closed chest massage technique.

DEFIBRILLATION

In 1774, the first case of resuscitation using electricity occurred. Sophia Greenhill, a child, fell from a window and was pronounced dead by physicians, but was revived by a layman who applied electric shocks to her thorax (Fig. 1). Dr. Charles Kite received a prize from the Royal Humane Society in 1788 for an instrument that may have been the first DC defibrillator. The instrument consisted of a Leyden jar to hold an electric charge and insulated brass electrodes for delivery of the shock anywhere on the body (Fig. 2).

By 1800, both electric shocks and ventilation were well-known resuscitative techniques. One such device combining these techniques is shown in Figure 3.

Mr. SQUIRES, OF SOHO, COMMUNICATED TO THE Rev. Mr. SOWDEN and Dr. HAWES.

ELECTRICITY RESTORED VITALITY.

ONE PART OF OUR BENEVOLENT DESIGN IS TO MANIFEST THE POSSIBILITY OF RECOVERY IN THE VARIOUS INSTANCES OF SUDDEN DEATH, WHERE THE VITAL POWERS ARE SUSPENDED, WITHOUT ANY ESSENTIAL INJURY TO THE FRAME. THIS EXTRAORDINARY RELATION OF RESUSCITATION ALSO MANIFESTS THE ADMIRABLE POWERS OF THE ELECTRICAL SHOCK; WHICH WE WOULD EARNESTLY RECOMMEND IN ALL CASES OF SUSPENDED ANIMATION.

SOPHIA GREENHILL, on Thursday last, fell out of a one-pair-of stairs window, and was taken up by a man to all appearance dead. The surgeons at the *Middlesex Hospital*, and an APOTHECARY, declared that nothing could be done for the child.—Mr. SQUIRES, tried the effects of electricity.—Twenty minutes elapsed before he could apply the shock, which he gave to various parts of the body in vain;—but, upon transmitting a few shocks through the THORAX, he perceived a *small pulsation*; in a few minutes the child began to breathe with great difficulty, and after some time she vomited.—A kind of stupor, occasioned by the depression of the cranium, remained for several days, but, by the proper means being used, her health was restored.

Figure 1. The first successful reversal of apparent death by electroshock took place in 1774. This singular incident secured for the resuscitationist, Mr. Squires, a niche in the archives of medical history. However, he was never heard from again after that brief moment of glory. (From Schechter DC: Early experience with resuscitation by means of electricity. Surgery *69*:360, 1971. Reprinted with permission.)

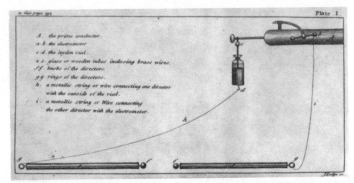

Figure 2. Dr. Kite's apparatus for resuscitation by means of electricity (1788). Parts of the apparatus include: *A*, the prime conductor; *a–b*, the electrometer; *c–d*, the Leyden vial; *e–e*, glass or wooden tubes enclosing brass wires; *f–f*, knobs of the directors; *g–g*, rings of the directors; *h*, a metallic string or wire connecting one director with the outside of the vial; *i*, a metallic string or wire connecting the other director with the electrometer. (From Payne JP: On the resuscitation of the apparently dead. Ann R Coll Surg Engl *45*:98, 1969. Redrawn; used with permission of the publisher.)

CONVERGENCE OF MODERN METHODS OF RESUSCITATION

Mouth-to-mouth ventilation was the first element of modern resuscitation to be refined. By 1954, Elam and others had established that mouth-to-mouth ventilation effectively reoxygenated the blood and restored normal carbon dioxide levels. Two years later, Elam and Safar compared the effectiveness of manual methods with the mouth-to-mouth method, showed the superiority of the latter, and demonstrated the necessity of maintaining a patent airway. By 1958, mouth-to-mouth resuscitation had substantially displaced the Nielsen method and others as the preferred technique for artificial respiration.

Electrotherapy and defibrillation techniques were also advanced. Beck performed the first successful open chest debrillation using AC current of the human heart in 1947. By 1948, development of closed chest defibrillation had begun, and in 1955, the first successful external defibrillation was accomplished by Paul Zoll and colleagues.

External cardiac compression, the third element in modern cardiopulmonary resuscitation, was rediscovered and developed by Kouwenhoven and associates during research on external cardiac defibrillation. By 1960, external cardiac compressions had been applied to 20 patients and had been attempted both with and without artificial respirations (including mouth-to-mouth).

External cardiac compression and mouth-to-mouth respiration were combined in the early 1960s, thus forming CPR as it is known

MILESTONES IN THE HISTORY OF RESUSCITATION

Date	Ventilation	Chest Compression	Defibrillation
1745	First reported case of mouth-to-mouth respiration (Tossach)		
1774			First resuscitation with electricity (Squires)
1778			Dr. Kite develops first direct current defibrillator
1796		Herholdt and Rafn describe chest compressions	
1858		First reported case of external heart massage (Balassa)	
1859			Friedburg demonstrates use of defibrillation in restoring heart rhythm
1874		Schiff establishes physiologic basis of heart massage	
1900			Prevost and Batteli describe electric shock in treatment of ventricular fibrillation
1901		First resuscitation using direct cardiac massage (Igelsrud)	
1947			First successful open chest defibrillation with direct current (Beck)
1954–56	Safar, Elam, and associates develop mouth-to-mouth methods		1955: First successful external defibrillation with alternating current defibrillator (Zoll)
1954–58		Development of external cardiac compression techniques (Kouwenhoven and associates)	
Early 1960s	Modern technique of CPR established: Combination of mouth-to-mouth resuscitation and external cardiac compressions (Kouwenhoven and associates)		DC defibrillators developed
1970s			Automatic implantable defibrillator developed
1980s			Automatic external defibrillator developed

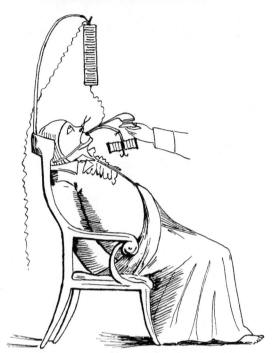

Figure 3. Reanimation chair invented by Richard Reece (1824): "The patient is extended on a 'reanimation chair,' the nostrils closed with forceps, and cotton tampons [put] in the ears. Air is pushed by bellows into a silver cannula in the larynx. Another inflexible metallic tube is inserted in the gullet. This is then rinsed with ether or any other stimulating fluid that may be thought proper. Concurrently (. . . and with seeming disregard for the risk of flame), one wire of a galvanic batter is fastened to the esophageal conduit, while the other is 'successively made to touch different parts of the external surface of the body, particularly about the regions of the hear the diaphragm . . . the neck . . .'" (From Schechter DC: Early experienc with resuscitation by means of electricity. Surgery 69:360, 1971. Reprinte with permission.)

today. CPR is effective, but by itself cannot maintain a patient who has suffered sudden cardiac death. CPR can "buy time" and sustain life until more definitive therapy—especially defibrillation and emergency medicines—becomes available.

REFERENCES

1. Hearne T: The history of cardiopulmonary resuscitation. In Eisenberg MS, Bergner L, Hallstrom AP (eds): Sudden Cardiac Death in the Community. New York, Praeger, 1984, pp. 17–28.
2. Kouwenhoven WB, Jude JR, Knickerbocker GG: Closed chest cardiac massage. JAMA 173:1064, 1960.

1

THE PATIENT IN SUDDEN CARDIAC ARREST

Every death ultimately is a cardiac arrest. However, the term *cardiac arrest* generally refers to unexpected loss of pulse and blood pressure resulting from heart disease. Even more specific is the term *sudden cardiac death*, defined as death by underlying heart disease occurring without symptoms or with symptoms of less than an hour's duration. Heart disease is the leading cause of death among adults in the United States, accounting for three quarters of a million deaths per year. Approximately two thirds, or 400,000 of these deaths, occur suddenly—frequently in individuals without known heart disease, and often in individuals in their most active years. The economic loss is immense, approaching 75 billion dollars per year.

EPIDEMIOLOGY OF OUT-OF-HOSPITAL SUDDEN CARDIAC DEATH

The approximate incidence of out-of-hospital sudden cardiac death is 1/1000 per year. The average age is 65 years (men, 63; women, 68), and men outnumber women by 3 to 1. There appears to be no seasonal or day of week association with cardiac arrest. There is, however, an association with the time of day. Fewer cardiac arrests occur during sleeping hours than at other times. Sleep may be protective or it may merely delay recognition of a cardiac arrest event.

Most out-of-hospital cardiac arrests (75%) occur in the patient's home.

RHYTHM ASSOCIATED WITH SUDDEN CARDIAC DEATH

The majority of cardiac arrests in the community are associated with ventricular fibrillation. Approximately 60% of patients with sudden cardiac death are found to be in ventricular fibrillation. (These rhythms are determined approximately 8–10 minutes after collapse, so the actual percentage of patients in ventricular fibrillation may be higher, owing to the delay in rhythm detection.) Other rhythms associated with sudden cardiac death include ventricular tachycardia, asystole, idioventricular rhythm, and sinus rhythm with electromechanical association.

Table 1–1. CARDIAC CAUSES OF SUDDEN DEATH IN ADULTS

Coronary atherosclerotic heart disease (accounts for the majority of deaths)
Coronary artery spasm
Coronary artery embolism
Valvular heart disease—primarily aortic stenosis and mitral valve prolapse
Cardiomyopathy, including idiopathic hypertrophic subaortic stenosis
Myocarditis
Bacterial endocarditis
Conduction defects—Wolff-Parkinson-White syndrome; prolonged QT
    syndrome; complete AV block
Cardiac tumors
Aortic dissection
Drug toxicity—quinidine syncope; digitalis toxicity

ETIOLOGY

The causes of sudden cardiac death are many. Table 1–1 lists the cardiac causes of sudden cardiac death in adults. Autopsy studies indicate that three quarters of patients with sudden cardiac death have significant atherosclerotic heart disease, usually involving major pathologic changes in two or three coronary arteries.

RISK FACTORS

Risk factors associated with sudden cardiac death are the same as those associated with the development of atherosclerotic heart disease, namely, hypertension, cigarette smoking, hypercholesterolemia, diabetes, male sex. The majority of individuals with sudden cardiac death have a history of atherosclerotic heart disease. Data from Seattle demonstrate that patients resuscitated from out-of-hospital ventricular fibrillation usually had prior manifestations of cardiovascular disease. Cobb and associates have shown a history of myocardial infarction, angina, congestive heart failure, and/or hypertension was present in 78% of patients who were resuscitated from sudden cardiac death. For the remaining 22%, cardiac arrest was the first manifestation of cardiovascular disease.

Clinical risk factors associated with sudden cardiac death include the following:

1. Ventricular ectopy (especially complex ventricular premature depolarizations), Lown class 3 or greater, in patients with cardiovascular disease (Fig. 1–1).

2. Extensive coronary artery narrowing.

3. Abnormal left ventricular function—for example, decreased ejection fraction, dyskinetic left ventricular wall motion.

4. Electrocardiographic abnormalities, such as prolonged QT intervals or repolarization abnormalities.

The sensitivity and specificity of these clinical predictors throughout the general population are not well defined, since most studies have been performed only on selected high-risk populations. Thus, the applicability to the general population, as well as the difficulty in performing some of these studies, limits widespread use. Furthermore, even if these clinical predictors were shown to be highly sensitive and specific, they would not be able to predict *when* the cardiac arrest would occur. There is, unfortunately, no unique or practical combination of recognizable risk factors that accurately identify patients who are at immediate risk of sudden cardiac death.

PATHOPHYSIOLOGY

It is not clear what mechanisms are responsible for sudden cardiac arrest or the initiation of ventricular fibrillation, the most common rhythm associated with sudden cardiac death. Numerous explanations of sudden cardiac death have been suggested, includ-

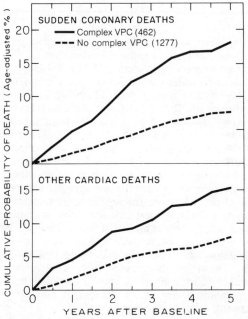

Figure 1–1. Mortality related to complex ventricular premature contractions (VPC) identified in 1 hour of ambulatory monitoring in patients with prior myocardial infarction. Premature beats were considered complex if they were multiform or repetitive, or if bigeminy or R on T was present. (From Ruberman W, Weinblatt E, Goldberg JD, et al: Ventricular premature complexes and sudden death after myocardial infarction. Circulation *64*:297, 1981. Reprinted with permission.)

Table 1–2. SYNDROMES OF SUDDEN CARDIAC DEATH

	Infarct	Ischemia	Electric
Pathophysiology	Infarcted area causes pump failure or may lead to rhythm disturbance	Ischemic area may trigger rhythm disturbance	Rhythm disturbance triggered by poorly understood causes
Percentage of sudden cardiac deaths	20–30%	Unknown	Unknown
Autopsy	Coronary artery occlusion with resultant myocardial infarct	Evidence of ischemia	"Normal" heart— usually evidence of underlying coronary artery disease
Most common rhythm	Ventricular fibrillation	Ventricular fibrillation	Ventricular fibrillation
Warning prior to collapse	Minutes to hours	Minutes	None or seconds
Mortality within 1 year after discharge	5%	Unknown	30%

ing ischemia, electrolyte imbalances, platelet abnormalities, psychological stress, and neurochemical transmitters.

Although coronary atherosclerotic heart disease is present in most patients with sudden cardiac arrest, only a minority of patients appear to have had an acute myocardial infarction associated with sudden cardiac death. Data from Cobb and associates demonstrate that approximately 20% of patients who were resuscitated and admitted to the hospital following out-of-hospital ventricular fibrillation had electrocardiographic evidence of acute transmural myocardial infarction. Almost half had ST-T wave changes; a smaller percentage had a myocardial infarction of indeterminate age; and approximately 25% had no electrocardiographic changes at all.

The lack of consistent electrocardiographic findings among patients resuscitated from sudden cardiac deaths suggests that several pathophysiologic syndromes may exist (see Table 1–2). Based upon prodromal symptoms, pathologic findings, and prognosis, it is possible to define one sudden cardiac death syndrome associated with primary electrical disturbance, another associated with ischemia, and a third connected with myocardial infarction. As etiologic mechanisms are better defined, it may be possible to characterize still more syndromes.

DETERMINANTS OF SURVIVAL FROM OUT-OF-HOSPITAL CARDIAC ARREST

Many factors determine whether an individual survives or dies following cardiac arrest. Factors that help to determine whether resuscitation will be successful can be categorized as fate factors and program factors. *Fate factors* are those related to the patients' individual characteristics or to chance, and include age, prior medical condition, presence of pathophysiologic conditions, cardiac rhythm, and whether or not the collapse was witnessed by others. A patient whose collapse was unwitnessed or who has rhythms other than ventricular fibrillation has a small likelihood of being resuscitated. *Program factors* are those determined by the configuration of the emergency care system and include type of service, whether or not a bystander initiates CPR, time from collapse to CPR, and time from collapse to definitive care. The factors most predictive of outcome are (a) time from collapse to CPR and (b) time from collapse to definitive care. The importance of these factors suggests the reason for the success of emergency systems utilizing combined EMT and paramedic personnel.

FATE FACTORS

Age and Sex

The average age of cardiac arrest patients is 65 years. Patients discharged following out-of-hospital cardiac arrest are an average of 61 years compared to 66 years for patients not surviving. There is no relationship of sex to admission or discharge.

Prior Medical Condition

Previous myocardial infarction or a history of congestive heart failure is associated with lower rates of survival from cardiac arrest.

Witnessed Collapse

In a witnessed cardiac arrest, a bystander sees or hears the collapse of the patient and responds immediately. In an unwitnessed cardiac arrest, the patient is discovered after collapse and therefore the time since collapse is unknown. As would be expected, patients whose collapse is witnessed have a much better survival rate than those whose collapse was unwitnessed.

Cardiac Rhythm

Patients in ventricular fibrillation or ventricular tachycardia have a much higher likelihood of admission and discharge than patients in other rhythms. In King County, Washington, ventricular fibrillation is the most common rhythm associated with cardiac arrest (58%; see Table 1–3). Of patients in ventricular fibrillation, 31% were discharged. Ventricular tachycardia, representing a much smaller number of cases (only 2% of the overall cases), also had a high likelihood of resuscitation, with 46% discharged. Patients with

Table 1–3. CARDIAC RHYTHM AND OUTCOME FOR PARAMEDIC-TREATED CASES

Rhythm (upon arrival)	Number (%)	Discharged (%)
Ventricular fibrillation	1238 (58%)	385 (31%)
Ventricular tachycardia	50 (2%)	23 (46%)
Asystole	576 (27%)	11 (2%)
Idioventricular	162 (8%)	5 (3%)
Other or unknown	125 (6%)	19 (15%)
Total	2151	443 (21%)

(Source: Center for Evaluation of Emergency Medical Services, Emergency Medical Services Division, King County Health Department, Seattle, WA.)

asystole and idioventricular rhythms had very poor outcomes (2% and 3% discharged, respectively).

PROGRAM FACTORS

Type of Service

Numerous studies have documented improved outcomes from cardiac arrest with paramedic care as compared with basic emergency medical technician (EMT) care. The improvement is explained by the paramedic's ability to provide definitive care at the scene as opposed to having to transport the patient to the hospital for definitive care, as basic EMTs must do. New programs that allow EMTs to defibrillate have improved survival from ventricular fibrillation.

Bystander Initiation of CPR

Initiation of CPR by bystanders at the scene improves outcome. As documented in Table 1–4, patients who received bystander CPR had higher discharge rates than those who did not receive bystander CPR.

Time from Collapse to Initiation of CPR

A short time between collapse and initiation of CPR is associated with successful outcome. In King County, Washington, when CPR was initiated in less than 4 minutes from collapse, 32% of the patients were discharged, compared with 17% of patients for whom CPR was initiated at 4 minutes or later.

Time from Collapse to Definitive Care

A significant linear relationship exists between outcome and the time from collapse to definitive care. In King County, Washington, when time to definitive care was less than 6 minutes, 37% were

Table 1–4. CONTROLLED STUDIES OF SURVIVAL (DISCHARGED FROM HOSPITAL ALIVE) FROM OUT-OF-HOSPITAL CARDIAC ARREST: BYSTANDER CPR COMPARED WITH DELAYED CPR*

Location/System[†]	Witnessed	Rhythm[‡]	Response Time	No.[§]	% (No.) Discharged From Hospital Alive
Oslo, EMTs only	Not reported	Not reported	Median "driving time" = 8 min	BYS CPR = 75 Delayed CPR = 556	36% (27) 8% (43)
Birmingham, AL, paramedics only	Implied yes	VF or VT	>5 min from call to arrival	BYS CPR = 7 Medic CPR = 12	86% (6) 50% (6)
Seattle, EMTs and paramedics	76% overall were witnessed	VF only	Mean = 3 min from dispatch to arrival	BYS CPR = 109 EMT CPR = 207	43% (47) 21% (43)
Winnipeg, Manitoba, EMTs only	Not reported	VF or VT	<10 min from call to arrival for only 12% of cases	BYS CPR = 65 EMT CPR = 161	25% (16) 5% (8)
Iceland, EMTs only	Not reported	All rhythms (42% = VF)	Mean = 7.3 min from call to arrival	BYS CPR = 38 EMT CPR = 84	42% (16) 6% (5)
Vancouver, EMTs and paramedics	77% overall were witnessed	All rhythms	Not reported	BYS CPR = 43 Delayed CPR = 272	21% (9) 6% (17)
Los Angeles, paramedics	41% overall were witnessed	All rhythms VF only	Mean = 5.0 min from call to arrival	BYS CPR = 93 Medic CPR = 150 BYS CPR = 45 Medic CPR = 70	22% (20) 5% (7) 27% (12) 6% (4)
King County, WA, EMTs and paramedics	Not reported	All rhythms	Mean = 6 min from collapse to EMT arrival	BYS CPR = 108 EMT CPR = 379	23% (25) 12% (45)
Pittsburgh, paramedics	Not reported	VF/VT only	Mean = 6.0 min dispatch to arrival	BYS CPR = 25 Medic CPR = 59	24% (6) 7% (4)

*CPR indicates cardiopulmonary resuscitation.
†EMTs indicates emergency medical technicians, or trained first responders.
‡VF indicates ventricular fibrillation; VT, ventricular tachycardia.
§BYS indicates bystander.
(From Cummins RO, Eisenberg MS: Prehospital cardiopulmonary resuscitation: is it effective? JAMA 253:2408, 1985. Reprinted with permission.)

13

Table 1–5. SURVIVAL RATES FROM CARDIAC ARREST RELATED TO THE PROMPTNESS OF INITIATION OF CPR AND DEFINITIVE CARE

		Time from Collapse to Delivery of Care		
		<8 min	8–16 min	>16 min
Time from Collapse to CPR	<4 min	43%	19%	10%
	4–8 min	27%	19%	6%
	>8 min		7%	0%

(From Eisenberg MS, Bergner L, Hallstrom A: JAMA *241*:1905, 1979. Reprinted with permission.)

discharged. When time to definitive care was greater than 14 minutes, 11% were discharged.

Time to CPR Combined with Time to Definitive Care

The two variables, time to CPR and time to definitive care, are interactively predictive of survival, and multivariate analysis shows them to be the most important program factors. Table 1–5 shows the relationship of outcome to these two times.

THE TIERED RESPONSE SYSTEM

Success of Utilizing EMTs and Paramedics

The two program factors most predictive of survival—time from collapse to CPR and time from collapse to definitive care—explain the reason for the success of emergency systems utilizing combined EMT and paramedic personnel. An emergency vehicle staffed with EMTs can arrive at the scene rapidly and begin CPR often within 4 minutes of collapse; this is the first component necessary for successful resuscitation. A second emergency vehicle staffed with paramedics can arrive several minutes later and provide definitive care; this is the second component necessary for successful resuscitation. The combination of these two factors, rapid onset of CPR and rapid provision of definitive care, is the essence of a successful out-of-hospital emergency care system for cardiac arrest.

CARDIAC ARREST IN THE HOSPITAL

The factors associated with successful resuscitation in the hospital are similar to those just discussed for cardiac arrest in the community. Patients who have ventricular fibrillation associated with the cardiac arrest fare much better than patients in other rhythms. Patients with witnessed or monitored arrests (generally those in coronary or intensive care units) have a higher survival rate than patients with unmonitored cardiac arrest. Most cases of in-hospital cardiac arrest are caused by underlying heart disease.

The number of successful in-hospital resuscitations roughly parallels the statistics seen with out-of-hospital resuscitation. Table 1–6 summarizes data from several studies of in-hospital cardiac arrest. The two most recent studies, from New York and Boston, are remarkable for their similarity in percentage initially resuscitated and percentage discharged from hospital. Bedell found that patients with pneumonia, hypotension, renal failure, cancer, or a home-bound lifestyle before hospitalization were less likely to be resuscitated. None of the patients with pneumonia and none in whom resuscitation took longer than 30 minutes were discharged. Age was not associated with likelihood of resuscitation.

TYPES OF CARDIAC ARREST

The term cardiac arrest merely describes a calamitous event in cardiac function and provides no indication as to etiology. As noted earlier, most cardiac arrests occurring out-of-hospital are caused by underlying heart disease, primarily atherosclerotic heart disease. A minority of out-of-hospital arrests (approximately 25%) are caused by noncardiac disease. The etiologies of noncardiac cardiac arrest include trauma, cancer, respiratory diseases, suicide, overdoses and poisonings, sudden infant death syndrome, and many other causes of death. In-hospital cardiac arrests are also predominately due to underlying heart disease; however, a fair proportion of cardiac arrests are the result of cancer, respiratory and neurologic disorders, and surgical complications.

Use of the term *cardiac arrest* implies that the event was sudden and presumably unexpected in nature. After all, every death ultimately involves cardiac arrest. Perhaps a better term would be *sudden cardiac arrest*, or *sudden cardiac death*. Including the word "sudden" indicates the unexpected nature of the event. The implication when using the term cardiac is that the cause of death was cardiac in nature. Because of these problems in terminology, we recommend the following classification, which may lead to more precision in the description of cardiac arrest:

Sudden Cardiac Arrest or Sudden Cardiac Death: Death caused by underlying heart disease occurring suddenly or within 1 hour of symptoms.

Cardiac Arrest: Death caused by underlying heart disease without reference to suddenness; a more general term encompassing all deaths due to underlying heart disease.

Circulatory Arrest: Death due to medical causes other than heart disease. Usually death does not occur suddenly and is preceded by

Table 1–6. SURVIVAL FROM CARDIAC ARREST AMONG HOSPITALIZED PATIENTS

Location	Reference	Number	% Resuscitated	% Discharged	Average Age	Long-Term Survival of Patients Discharged
Charlottesville	15	368	25%	8%	54*	—
Hartford	16	237	41%	22%	66*	—
Montreal	17	1204	—	19%	65	74% at 1 yr
Washington, D.C.	18	734	42%	4%	59	—
Buffalo	19	123	—	8%	70	—
Dayton	20	1073	57%	24%	60	75% at 1 yr
New York	21	226	41%	14%	70	70% at 6 mo
Boston	22	294	44%	14%	70	80% at 5 mo

*Estimated from available data.

symptoms of variable duration depending on the underlying disease.

Traumatic Circulatory Arrest: Death due to trauma.

THE SPECTRUM OF ARRESTS

Cardiac Arrest

In sudden cardiac arrest or cardiac arrest in general, the primary disorder lies in the heart; thus, when the heart's contractions cease, blood pressure and pulse fall to zero. Sometimes, agonal respirations may continue for seconds or even up to a few minutes. These respirations are not normal respirations and may be characterized more as gasping and very slow respiratory efforts. Agonal respirations probably occur because oxygenated blood pooled in the midbrain allows stimulation of the respiratory centers for a short while.

Respiratory Arrest

Cessation of cardiac contractions may be due to any cause ranging from primary dysrhythmias to trauma-induced hypovolemia. In some situations the heart may still be contracting, but respirations may have ceased and/or hypotension may be present. If respirations cease but the heart is still contracting, the term respiratory arrest should be used. This situation is usually encountered in patients with overdoses, respiratory disease, metabolic disease, and a variety of medical conditions. Respiratory arrest is rarely caused by underlying heart disease. In respiratory arrest, the primary disorder is in the respiratory system (or a result of hypoxia); thus, respirations cease before cardiac contractions cease. Usually in respiratory arrest, diminution and cessation of cardiac contractions will occur within several minutes. Therefore, all respiratory arrests will become circulatory arrests if left untreated.

Near Arrests

Near arrests refer to situations in which the heart is still contracting but in an ineffective manner, resulting in severe loss of blood pressure. The pulse may be thready or absent, and respirations often cease. Consciousness is usually lost in near-arrest situations. Near-arrest situations occur in a variety of clinical settings, some of the more common examples being cardiogenic shock, severe pulmonary edema, sepsis, and kidney failure. When the blood pressure falls below 60 mm Hg palpable, cardiopulmonary resuscitation is indicated. A rough rule of thumb is that the carotid pulse can be felt at 60 mm Hg systolic, the femoral pulse at 70 mm Hg, and the radial pulse at 80 mm Hg. Typically, in near-arrest situations, the heart will be contracting as can be seen on the ECG monitor, the pulse will be lost, and the blood pressure will be extremely low and detected only with the aid of a Doppler.

ANTICIPATING AND PREVENTING CARDIAC ARREST

Often cardiac arrest cannot be anticipated. For example, many cases of sudden cardiac arrest occur without warning or with only the briefest of premonitory symptoms. Nonetheless, there are situations in which action can be taken to lessen the chances of cardiac arrest. The most frequently encountered clinical situation in which preventive measures may play a role is in the management of myocardial infarction.

When myocardial infarction is suspected, therapy should be prompt and vigorous. Cardiac rhythms should be monitored continuously. Oxygen should be administered, preferably by nasal prongs at a low flow in an alert patient. Management of pain should be vigorous, with the goal being the elimination of complaints of pain. Morphine is the analgesic of choice. Usually small IV increments of 2–5 mg are given q 5 min until relief occurs. Nitroglycerin (sublingual, paste) is effective in angina, but often will not eliminate the pain of infarction. Intravenous nitroglycerin is often effective in managing the pain of infarction, but should not be used in place of morphine. Depending on the type of infarction and the duration of symptoms, thrombolytic therapy may be considered (assuming there are no contraindications).

An important therapeutic step is the use of prophylactic lidocaine to prevent the occurrence of ventricular fibrillation. Lidocaine should be used in patients *highly* suspected of myocardial infarction and probably should *not* be used prophylactically in patients with a low probability of myocardial infarction. When used for primary prophylaxis, lidocaine should be given regardless of the presence of PVCs. In other words, PVCs are not needed to justify prophylactic lidocaine if infarction is highly suspected. A variety of

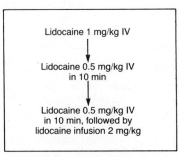

Figure 1–2. Prophylaxis of VF in patients suspected of myocardial infarction with no ventricular ectopy. (See Chapter 10 for treatment of ventricular ectopy.)

methods may be used to provide prophylaxis. In the method, outlined in Figure 1–2, a loading dose of 1 mg/kg is given IV, with additional 0.5 mg/kg doses given every 10 minutes to a loading dose of 2 mg/kg. After a loading dose, an intravenous infusion of 2 mg/min is begun. With prolonged administration—i.e., beyond 24–48 hours—lidocaine blood levels increase, and the infusion should be lowered or blood levels monitored. (See Chapter 10 for treatment of ventricular ectopy.)

OUTCOMES FOLLOWING CARDIAC ARREST

Most studies reporting neurologic outcomes, morbidity, and mortality following cardiac arrest have focused on out-of-hospital events. This is primarily because cardiac arrest in hospitalized patients is complicated by co-morbidity, thus making it difficult to demonstrate the independent consequences of the cardiac arrest. The following discussion is confined exclusively to out-of-hospital cardiac arrest.

Neurologic Recovery

Once initial resuscitation occurs, the clinician as well as family members must confront the very real possibility either of death occurring during hospitalization or of recovery with neurologic deficits.

The likelihood of death occurring in the hospital following out-of-hospital resuscitation is approximately 50%. Most deaths are the result of anoxic brain damage or cardiovascular shock.

Longstreth and colleagues reported on the likelihood of neurologic recovery following out-of-hospital cardiac arrest and admission to the hospital. The probability of awakening decreased with each day of coma, and the length of coma was associated with the degree of neurologic recovery. Two thirds of the patients awakening within hours of admission had full neurologic recovery. Of the patients who were comatose for 24 hours after admission, 40% regained consciousness. Of the patients awakening after 4 days, 80% had significant motor and cognitive deficits. Longstreth developed a score to calculate the probability of awakening. The score is calculated at the time of admission and is determined by the motor response, pupillary light response, spontaneous eye movements, and blood glucose level. Table 1–7 shows how the score is calculated. Patients with high scores have a very high probability of regaining consciousness.

Long-Term Survival

Studies from several communities reporting long-term survival following out-of-hospital cardiac arrest are shown in Table 1–8.

Table 1–7. RULE TO CALCULATE PROBABILITY OF AWAKENING SCORES

Motor Response	+	3 × Pupillary Light Response	+	Spontaneous Eye Movements	+	Blood Glucose Level on Admission
0 — Absent		0 — absent		0 — absent		0 — >300 mg/dl
1 — Extensor posturing		1 — present		1 — present		1 — <300 mg/dl
2 — Flexor posturing						
3 — Nonposturing						
4 — Withdrawal or localizing						

Interpretation:

Score	Probability of Awakening
0,1,2	<5
3,4	<25%
5,6,7	<75%
8,9	>95%
Over 4	>80%
4 or less	<16%

Modified, with permission, from Longstreth WT, Inui TS, Cobb MK: Neurologic recovery after out-of-hospital cardiac arrest. Ann Intern Med 98(Part 1):588, 1983; and from Longstreth WT, Diehr P, Inui TS: Prediction of awakening after out-of-hospital cardiac arrest. N Engl J Med 1983;308:1378, 1983.

Table 1–8. STUDIES REPORTING LONG-TERM SURVIVAL FOLLOWING RESUSCITATION, AND DISCHARGE FROM OUT-OF-HOSPITAL CARDIAC ARREST

Location	Reference	No. of Patients	Type of Patient*	Long-Term Survival: Percent Alive at			
				1 yr	2 yr	3 yr	4 yr
Oslo, Norway	30	94	All patients, including trauma	—	80		—
Miami	31	42	VF†		Mean survival: 31 months		
Minneapolis	32	47	All patients‡	85			
Michigan & Ohio	33	142	All patients	82§	50		48§
Seattle	34	406	VF	74	66§	55§	50
King County, WA	35	276	Cardiac arrest owing to heart disease	76	64	55	49

*Unless indicated, trauma patients are excluded.

†VF = Ventricular Fibrillation

‡Only ambulatory patients were followed long-term.

§Estimated from data contained in article.

(Modified, with permission, from Eisenberg M, Bergner L, Hallstrom A (eds): Sudden Cardiac Death in the Community. Philadelphia, Praeger, 1984.)

Table 1–9. STUDIES REPORTING MORBIDITY OF PATIENTS AFTER RESUSCITATION AND DISCHARGE FROM OUT-OF-HOSPITAL CARDIAC ARREST

Location	Reference	No.	Type of Patient*	Morbidity
Oslo	30	94	All patients, including trauma	21% with mental impairment
Miami	31	42	Ventricular fibrillation	60% pre-arrest status 28% some impairment but could function at home 12% severe neurologic deficit
Minneapolis	32	83	All patients	60% full mental function 40% chronic care facility
Aahrus	39	36	All patients	22% residual brain damage 6% institutionalized
St. Paul	40	25	All patients	64% excellent recovery 32% good recovery 4% poor recovery
Denver	41	20†	All patients	53% independent living 32% returned to work
Seattle	34	21	Ventricular fibrillation	57% normal or slight impairment of exercise capacity
Seattle and King County, WA	1	426	Ventricular fibrillation	9% chronic care facility; most returned to pre-arrest status

*Unless indicated, trauma patients are excluded.
†20 to 28 patients still alive 3½ years following out-of-hospital cardiac arrest.
(Adapted from Bergner L, Eisenberg MS: J Cardiovasc Med 8:1223, 1983.)

In studies from King County, Washington, 276 of 302 cardiac arrest patients (due to heart disease) discharged from the hospital were followed to determine long-term survival. The probability of survival following discharge was 76% at 1 year, and 49% at 4 years. An age- and sex-matched "normal" group had a survival of 80% at 4 years, and a comparable group of discharged MI patients (without cardiac arrest) had a 4-year survival of 66%.

MEASURES OF MORBIDITY

Characterizing the functional status of survivors is as important as defining the mortality experience. What is the residual damage, neurologic or otherwise, to a person, and what is the patient's capacity to return to a pre–cardiac arrest level of functioning? The difficulty with many studies describing morbidity lies in the methodology. Most studies are case series. Another problem is the vague and nonspecific characterizations of function. With these problems in mind, most studies report that a majority of patients, approximately 60%, achieve a good recovery and return to their pre-arrest level of function. Approximately 30% have moderate dysfunction, and 10% have significant impairment (Table 1–9). Among patients studied in King County who had been working prior to their cardiac arrest, a majority returned to work.

The overall prognosis following out-of-hospital cardiac arrest leaves much room for improvement. As shown in Table 1–10, for every 100 out-of-hospital cardiac arrests due to heart disease, 40 will be successfully resuscitated and admitted to hospital. Twenty will be discharged, 14 will be alive at 1 year, and of these, 9 will achieve their pre-arrest level of function. (These estimates are based upon data from King County, Washington.) These figures are from a community with an excellent pre-hospital emergency medical system. The experience in most other communities is much poorer. The only means to improve upon these figures is to provide CPR and definitive care (of which defibrillation is the most important component) as soon as possible.

Table 1–10. OUTCOMES FOLLOWING OUT-OF-HOSPITAL CARDIAC ARREST DUE TO HEART DISEASE*

Patient Status	Number of Patients
Out-of-hospital cardiac arrest due to heart disease (all rhythms)	100
Admitted to hospital	40
Discharged	20
Alive at 1 year post discharge	14
Achieve prehospital level of functioning	9

*Figures based upon data from Center for Evaluation of Emergency Medical Services, Emergency Medical Services Division, King County Health Department, Seattle, WA.

REFERENCES

Epidemiology

1. Eisenberg MS, Bergner L, Hallstrom A: Sudden Cardiac Death in the Community. New York, Praeger, 1984.
2. Lown B: Sudden cardiac death: The major challenge confronting contemporary cardiology. Am J Cardiol 43:313, 1979.
3. Kuller LH: Sudden death—definition and epidemiologic considerations. Prog Cardiovasc Dis 23:1, 1980.

Risk Factors

4. Cobb LA, Werner JA: Predictors and prevention of sudden cardiac death. In Hurst JW (ed): The Heart. New York, McGraw-Hill, 1982.
5. Ruberman W, Weinblatt E, Goldberg JD, et al: Ventricular premature beats and mortality after myocardial infarction. Circulation 64:297, 1981.
6. Cobb LA, Werner J, Trobough G: Sudden cardiac death. I. A decade's experience with out-of-hospital resuscitation. Mod Concepts Cardiovasc Dis 49:31, 1980.
7. Goldstein S, Landis JR, Leighton R, et al: Characteristics of the resuscitated out-of-hospital cardiac arrest victim with coronary heart disease. Circulation 64:977, 1981.

Out-of-Hospital Cardiac Arrest

8. Eisenberg MS, Bergner L, Hearne T: Out-of-hospital cardiac arrest: a review of major studies and a proposed uniform reporting system. Am J Publ Health 70:236, 1980.
9. Cobb LA, Baum RS, Alvarez H, et al: Resuscitation from out-of-hospital ventricular fibrillation: four-year follow-up. Circulation 51(Suppl III):223, 1975.
10. Lewis RP, Stang JM, Fulkerson PK, et al: Effectiveness of advanced paramedics in a mobile coronary care system. JAMA 241:1902, 1979.
11. Cobb LA, Werner JA, Trobaugh GB: Sudden cardiac death. 2. Outcome of resuscitation, management and future directions. Mod Concepts of Cardiovasc Dis (AHA) 6:37, 1980.
12. Eisenberg MS, Bergner L, Hallstrom A: Sudden Cardiac Death in the Community. New York, Praeger, 1984.
13. Cummins RO, Eisenberg MS: Prehospital cardiopulmonary resuscitation: is it effective? JAMA 253:2408, 1985.
14. Eisenberg M, Bergner L, Hallstrom A: Cardiac resuscitation in the community: the importance of rapid delivery of care and implications for program planning. JAMA 241:1905, 1979.

In-Hospital Cardiac Arrest

15. Hollingsworth JH: The results of cardiopulmonary resuscitation: a 3-year university hospital experience. Ann Intern Med 71:459, 1969.
16. Jeresaty RM, Godar TJ, Liss JP, et al: External cardiac resuscitation in a community hospital. Arch Intern Med 245:588, 1969.
17. Lemire JG, Johnson AL: Is cardiac resuscitation worthwhile: a decade of experience. N Engl J Med 286:970, 1972.
18. Peschin A, Coakley CS: A five-year review of 734 cardiopulmonary arrests. South Med J 63:506, 1970.
19. Saphir R: External cardiac massage: prospective analysis of 123 cases and review of the literature. Medicine 45:73, 1968.
20. DeBard ML: Cardiopulmonary resuscitation: analysis of six years experience and review of the literature. Ann Emerg Med 10:408, 1981.
21. Suljaga-Pechtel K, Goldberg E, Strickson P, et al: Cardiopulmonary resuscitation in a hospitalized population: prospective study of factors associated with outcome. Resuscitation 12:77, 1984.
22. Bedell SE, Delbanco TL, Cook EF, et al: Survival after cardiopulmonary resuscitation in the hospital. N Engl J Med 309:569, 1983.

Prophylaxis with Lidocaine

23. DeSilva RA, Hennekens CH, Lown B, et al: Lidocaine prophylaxis in acute myocardial infarction: an evaluation of randomized trials. Lancet 2:855, 1981.
24. Koster RW, Dunning AJ: Intramuscular lidocaine for prevention of lethal arrhythmias in the prehospital phase of acute myocardial infarction. N Engl J Med 313:1105, 1985.
25. Bethesda Conference Report, Thirteenth Bethesda Conference: Emergency Cardiac Care. Am J Cardiol 50:365, 1982.
26. Carruth JE, Silverman ME: Ventricular fibrillation complicating acute myocardial infarction: reasons against the routine use of lidocaine. Am Heart J 104:545, 1982.
27. Davison R, Parker M, Atkinson AJ: Excessive serum lidocaine levels during maintenance infusions: mechanisms and prevention. Am Heart J 104:203, 1982.

Long-Term Survival

28. Longstreth WT Jr, Inui TS, Cobb LA, et al: Neurologic recovery after out-of-hospital cardiac arrest. Ann Intern Med 98(Part I):588, 1983.
29. Longstreth WT Jr, Diehr P, Inui TS: Prediction of awakening after out-of-hospital cardiac arrest. N Engl J Med 308:1378, 1983.
30. Lund I, Skulburg A: Resuscitation of cardiac arrest outside hospitals: experience with a mobile intensive care unit in Oslo. Acta Anaesth Scand 53:13, 1973.
31. Liberthson RR, Nagel EL, Hirschman JS, et al: Prehospital ventricular fibrillation: prognosis and follow-up course. N Engl J Med 291:317, 1974.
32. Rockwold G, Sharma B, Ruiz E, et al: Follow-up of 514 consecutive patients with cardiopulmonary arrest outside the hospital. JACEP 8:216, 1979.
33. Goldstein S, Landis JR, Leighton R, et al: Characteristics of the resuscitated out-of-hospital cardiac arrest victim with coronary heart disease. Circulation 64:977, 1981.
34. Cobb LA, Werner JA, Trobaugh GB: Sudden cardiac death. I. A decade's experience with out-of-hospital resuscitation. Mod Concepts Cardiovasc Dis 49:31, 1980.
35. Eisenberg MS, Hallstrom AP, Bergner L: Long-term survival after out-of-hospital cardiac arrest. N Engl J Med 306:1340, 1982.
36. Kaplan EL, Meier P: Nonparametric estimation from incomplete observations. J Am Stat Assoc 53:457, 1958.
37. Kishpaugh KK, Ford MH, Castle CH, et al: Myocardial infarction: a five-year follow-up of patients. West J Med 134:1, 1981.
38. Cobb LA, Baum RS, Alvarez H, et al: Resuscitation from out-of-hospital ventricular fibrillation: 4 year follow-up. Circulation 52(Suppl III):223, 1975.
39. Wernberg M, Thomassen A: Prognosis after cardiac arrest occurring outside intensive care and coronary units. Acta Anaesth Scand 23:69, 1979.
40. Snyder BD, Loewenson RB, Gumnit RJ, et al: Neurologic prognosis after cardiopulmonary arrest. II. Level of consciousness. Neurology 30:52, 1980.
41. Earnest M, Yarnell PR, Merrill SL, et al: Long-term survival and neurologic status after resuscitation from out-of-hospital cardiac arrest. Neurology 30:1298, 1980.

2

CODE ORGANIZATION

A team approach with leadership, defined roles, and integration of tasks offers the best chance for a successful resuscitation.

The number and makeup of the members of a code team vary with the situation and institution. Regardless of the composition of the team, the lead member must be familiar with the tasks associated with each of the assigned roles. A team leader (TL) must be designated and clearly recognized by each member of the code team. The TL's task is to lead and coordinate the resuscitation team. The team members (TM) have the responsibility of supporting the TL and performing what is expected in their assigned roles.

Proper care dictates that management will move from basic life support (usually delivered by emergency medical technicians [EMTs]) to advanced life support (delivered by paramedics before arrival at the hospital or by physicians and nurses in emergency departments) to critical care units. Transfer periods via ambulance or to critical care units from emergency departments are critically vulnerable times.

PHASES IN CODE ORGANIZATION

A code proceeds through several phases: anticipation, entry, resuscitation, maintenance, family notification, transfer, and critique. While each patient is unique, the principles of each phase remain the same.

Phase I: Anticipation

A. Analyze prehospital data
B. Gather the team
C. State leadership
D. Delineate duties
E. Prepare and check equipment
F. Position oneself

In this section, we assume that resuscitation has begun outside the hospital and the emergency department has been notified. The TL's first task is to analyze critical data by radio or telephone. Based upon available information, the TL gathers the team, states leadership, and delineates duties. Airway control, chest massage, vascular access, record keeping, patient disrobing, medication

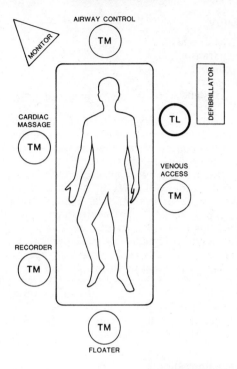

TL: Team Leader
TM: Team Member

Figure 2–1. Typical position of team leader and team members.

preparation, and delivery of specimens to the laboratory are basic assignments. Consultants must be alerted early. If needed, the trauma team, anesthesiologist, backup physicians, and nursing personnel are notified. Prehospital data analysis may dictate that O negative blood be present upon the patient's arrival. The TMs prepare and check equipment: laryngoscope lights are checked; ET/NT tubes appropriate for the patient's age and size are secured, and cuffs are tested; IVs are hung; procedure packs are placed (not opened unless prehospital data support this); the monitor-defibrillator is tested; the suction machine is turned on; and so on.

The TL and TMs position themselves contingent upon the physical makeup of the resuscitation room (Fig. 2–1). The TL has an overview of the resuscitation, without impeding the flow of movement or the view of other team members. For the TL this is frequently to the left or right of the patient's upper chest, with a clear view of the monitor. In many departments the monitor and defibrillator are combined and positioned next to the TL.

Phase II: Entry

A. Enter vital signs
B. Orderly transfer
C. ABC baseline
D. Brief history
E. New vital signs

Usually, the last prehospital vital signs (VS) are performed several minutes before arrival at the hospital, and this information should be given upon entry into the emergency department. The TL should receive this information directly from the EMTs or paramedics. Room access by ambulance stretcher must be optimal, allowing for the orderly transfer to the emergency department gurney on command of the TL. The TMs obtain a baseline of airway, breathing, circulation, and neuro status (level of consciousness, pupil size and response, motor lateralization). While this is being obtained, the paramedic-in-charge provides the TL with a brief history. This includes chief complaint, age, mechanism of injury, vital sign status, and pertinent physical findings and other information necessary to the resuscitation transfer. This may include IV needle size, volume of fluid and response, MAST suit pressure, known allergies, patient medications, estimation of blood loss at the scene, and rhythm interpretation. By this time the TMs are prepared to provide new vital signs.

Phase III: Resuscitation

A. Keep to the ABCs
B. Decisive, professional, unflappable
C. Information fed to the leader:
  1. Vital signs every 5 minutes or with change in patient's parameters
  2. On completion of procedures/medication
  3. Clarification
  4. Primary and secondary assessment information
  5. TL's own observations
D. Return to ABCs for:
  1. Treatment failure
  2. Unstable vital signs
  3. Prior to any procedures
  4. Routine and periodic
E. "Any suggestions"

It is imperative that the team keep to the ABCs. Avoid distractions. For example, airway control necessitates that the TM observe for chest wall excursions, facial color, and resistance to ventilation. The excitement of the event may easily distract any TM, but most critically those involved in the management and maintenance of the ABCs. In a short time many of these functions (i.e., ventilation and chest compressions) become fatiguing, and the TL must anticipate this problem.

The TL must be familiar with algorithms, management protocols, potential complications, responsibilities of TMs and means of communication. The more stressful the situation, the more calm the TL and TMs need to be. TMs react to the anxiety or calmness of the TL. Being decisive, professional, and unflappable are favorable TL traits. The TL must be prepared to transfer leadership at any time if he or she must respond to another critical problem.

Keep spectators out. Honor and respect the patient's right to privacy.

The resuscitation room must be sufficiently quiet for all to hear the TL's orders. The TL may find it necessary to reassert that one voice, and only one voice, should be heard above all others. Information fed to the TL is selective. Data on vital signs, including mental status, are concisely provided every 5 minutes or sooner if there is a significant change. On completion of any procedure or medication, a confirmatory brief statement is related to the TL, e.g., "Atropine 1 mg per central line completed"; "Chest tube in place and draining red blood approximately 200 cc per minute"; "ET tube in place, bilateral and equal breath sounds, ventilating at 24 per minute with 100% O_2."

TMs must request clarification on any orders or response to an order if any confusion exists. This should be stated in a well-focused fashion, e.g., "Repeat your last order"; "Is the order for epinephrine 1 mg per IV or ET tube?"

As primary and secondary assessment information accumulates, it is provided to the TL by TMs or recognized consultants. It is appropriate for the TL to provide an equally succinct overview of essential information periodically to the team. This enhances team effort and communication, restimulates anticipatory responses, reasserts leadership, serves as clarification, and reduces anxiety. At the same time, the TL's own observations are articulated, e.g., "Capillary perfusion is improved"; "PVCs are controlled; we'll continue the lidocaine drip as ordered."

Answers to treatment failures are usually found somewhere in the ABCs. If VSs remain unstable or deteriorate rapidly, recheck the ABCs. Frequently a correctable problem (such as an ET tube lodged in the right main stem bronchus, or jugular venous distension suggesting tamponade or pneumothorax) remains undetected.

Invasive procedures provide distractions. Prior to the procedure, rapidly recheck the ABCs to ensure that the optimal environment exists.

The TL should ask the team if there are any suggestions for management. This is appropriately asked with treatment failures, prior to transfer, and before terminating a code.

Phase IV: Maintenance

  A. Stabilize, fixate, and stay ahead
  B. Adrenalin rush subsides
  C. Vulnerable period
  D. Maintain team attention

Vital signs that are now stable were once not! To ensure stabilization, anticipation must remain acute. Once the patient is stabilized and the tension and excitement diminishes, the normal adrenalin rush of the team subsides. This may prove to be the most dangerously vulnerable period for patient and team alike. Reminders of this fact must be articulated by the TL while the TMs fixate IV lines on arm boards, and secure thoracostomy or ET tubes. The TL must, at all times, maintain team attention and stay ahead by troubleshooting potential problem areas and decoding subtle alterations in vital signs.

Phase V: Family Notification

  A. Appraisal and status
  B. Disposition

Responsibility to apprise the family of the situation falls to the TL or designate. Few guidelines exist. It is critical to (a) identify that the patient is indeed who he or she is thought to be, (b) establish the relationship of those present, (c) accurately restate the events leading up to the resuscitation, (d) emphasize that a thorough team effort was undertaken, and (e) briefly outline the patient's present condition. After allowing for appropriate emotional expression, the family is informed of the immediate disposition of the patient and the identity of those providers who will continue responsibility for care. A chaplain or social worker is an invaluable part of the team and should be present early on to provide support and clarification.

Statements concerning death should come from the TL or designate and are best articulated directly, e.g., "Despite the team's efforts, your father has died." Vague terminology such as "he's no longer with us" will only confuse and foster anger. One should not shy away from direct eye contact, physical comforting, or sharing of emotion. The family may wish to view the body. Prepare them for what to expect, as all tubes and invasive lines frequently remain in place in anticipation of a coroner's autopsy review.

In certain circumstances one will be called upon to clearly define brain death. Family consultation is required to determine the potential for harvesting organs for transplant. Expert consultation should be obtained immediately when protocols for transplant and brain death are not known.

Phase VI: Transfer

Team responsibility continues without abeyance and does not cease until a transfer to another location and another team has occurred (such as to the Critical Care Unit).

Phase VII: Critique

A. Critical responsibility
B. Grieving process
C. Education

Critique is a necessary responsibility of every team, no matter how brief, routine, or complex the code. If appropriate, feedback to prehospital personnel is provided at a later time. TMs will come away from any code with dissimilar feelings and reactions, based primarily on their prior code experiences, identification with the patient, sense of loss, performance anxiety or failure, and individual personalities. The grieving process must be attended to at this time. This process occurs not only with death but with anticipated death and patient loss of limb or function. Indeed, this is the most critical time to provide educational feedback to all team members, to discuss procedures or decisions to terminate the code, to explain the pathophysiology of the event and the TL's decision making, and to discuss possible improvements for the future.

REFERENCES

1. American Heart Association: Advanced Cardiac Life Support, Dallas, 1983.
2. American College of Surgeons, Committee on Trauma: Advanced Trauma Life Support Course for Physicians, Chicago, 1984.
3. Cassem NH, Hackett TP: The setting of intensive care. In Hackett TP, Cassem NH (eds): Massachusetts General Hospital Handbook of General Hospital Psychiatry. St. Louis, Mosby, 1978.

3

ADULT BASIC CARDIOPULMONARY RESUSCITATION

Basic cardiopulmonary resuscitation (CPR) is a core feature of advanced cardiac life support (ACLS). It should not be looked upon as just a task performed out-of-hospital by ambulance drivers, or in-hospital by medical students, nurses, or whoever happens to be present at a "code." Basic CPR skills provide the rescuer with a sequence of actions—a mental prioritization of what to do next—that can be repeatedly valuable in emergency practice. The sequence of one-rescuer CPR introduces and focuses many features of ACLS.

This chapter reviews the steps of basic CPR in detail, from the perspective of the ACLS team leader. It presents the rationale for many of the steps of basic CPR, and emphasizes those features that the ACLS team leader must monitor closely for proper performance. The ACLS team leader has the responsibility to be thoroughly familiar with basic CPR, not only in order to supervise and monitor the performance of others but also in preparation for that inevitable day when the ACLS team leader arrives "first on the scene" of a cardiac arrest.

Changes between the 1979 AHA Standards and Guidelines and the 1986 AHA Standards and Guidelines are noted and discussed.

MAJOR FEATURES OF BASIC CPR: The ABCs

Airway

1. Initial Assessment: Verify Unconsciousness. An unconscious person should always be considered to have respiratory arrest or cardiac arrest, or both, until proved otherwise. First, the clinical state of coma is verified by "shaking and shouting" the person suspected of having a cardiac arrest. This shaking and shouting maneuver distinguishes a person who is merely asleep or who has a depressed sensorium from one who is clinically comatose.

2. Call for Help. Once unresponsiveness is verified, the rescuer should immediately CALL FOR HELP. When another person responds, that individual should be directed to activate the emergency medical system.

Comment: To give priority to a CALL FOR HELP when unconsciousness is verified and, a few seconds later, to

ACTIVATION OF THE EMERGENCY MEDICAL SERVICE SYSTEM when pulselessness is determined, underscores the principle that *advanced* care, in the form of electrical defibrillation, definitive airway management, and intravenous pharmacology, must be brought to the patient as soon as possible. A rescuer should never forget that the prime chance for a successful resuscitation comes from decreasing the time from the onset of the arrest to the restoration of an effective spontaneous circulation. This means that additional people must be summoned, as quickly as possible, to assist the rescuer. When additional help arrives, they will be directed to assist with CPR, to get available ACLS equipment, to activate the resuscitation team (if in a hospital setting), or to activate the emergency medical system.

3. Appropriately Position the Victim. If the presumed arrest victim is not on a firm surface and supine, he or she must be rolled over as one unit, with the head, neck, and trunk maintained in a straight line, to stabilize the cervical spine. Do this by kneeling beside the person and placing one hand on the back of the head and neck; with the other hand roll the patient slowly toward you. This method must be strictly followed if there is any suspicion of cervical injury. If two people are available to turn a prone victim over, the second person should be positioned at the head of the patient and maintain jaw or head traction while the patient is turned. When the person is in bed, a firm support must be placed under the thoracic cage. A plywood board is kept for this purpose on most hospital units.

Comment: Physiologists dispute the mechanism of blood flow that occurs during the chest compressions of CPR. Some contend that the chest compressions squeeze the heart between the sternum and the vertebral bodies of the spine; others argue that the blood flow is produced by increased intrathoracic pressure. The important point here is that for chest compressions to be effective, regardless of the mechanism, the victim must be flat on his or her back on a firm surface, with the head no higher than the chest.

4. Appropriately Position the Rescuer. The most efficient position for a single rescuer is to kneel at the level of the victim's shoulders. In this position the rescuer can move from the mouth to the chest of the victim without moving the knees.

5. Open the Airway. As a first step, the mouth should be opened and the upper airway inspected for foreign objects, vomitus, or blood. If present, these should be removed with the fingers covered with gauze or a piece of cloth, or by turning the patient on the side, paying careful attention to the possibility of a cervical spine injury.

The American Heart Association recommends a combination of the head-tilt maneuver with the chin-lift maneuver as the best layperson method for opening the airway. Emergency professionals should also learn the jaw-thrust technique.

a. *Head tilt.* One hand is placed on the victim's forehead, and backward pressure is applied with the palm to tilt the head back. In many arrests this maneuver is sufficient to lift the back of the tongue and clear the airway.

b. *Chin lift.* Next, the fingers of the other hand are placed under the symphysis of the mandible. The chin is lifted forward until the teeth are barely touching, but the mouth is not completely closed. The thumb is not used, and the fingers must not press deeply into the soft tissue under the chin. The other hand remains against the forehead.

c. *Jaw thrust.* The rescuer stands or kneels at the head of the patient and grasps the mandible of the jaw with the fingertips while the hands are placed at the sides of the patient's face. The mandible is lifted forward. A position with the elbows on the stretcher or backboard is usually the most comfortable one for the rescuer. The jaw-thrust technique must be learned by all rescuers who may encounter patients with the combination of cervical spine injuries and respiratory compromise. It maintains a neutral position of the cervical spine while resuscitation attempts continue. This technique is used almost solely for trauma patients by out-of-hospital response teams.

Comment: At this point rescuers may encounter a common problem in the airway management of cardiac arrest victims—the victim is wearing dentures. With the exception of endotracheal intubation, all methods of airway management in basic and advanced life support work better if the cheeks, lips, and jaws are supported by well-fitted and in-place dentures. Unless the dentures are obviously loose and posing an airway obstruction problem themselves, they should NOT be removed.

Breathing

6. Assess Breathlessness. An assessment of the ability to move air is quickly made when the rescuer opens the airway with the head-tilt/chin-lift maneuvers, and then "looks, listens, and feels" for air movement. The "look, listen, and feel" technique is performed with the rescuer's head in one position, with the ear placed almost touching the patient's mouth and the face turned toward the victim's chest. The rescuer "listens and feels" for breathing with his or her ear, and simultaneously "looks" at the victim's chest for any respiratory movements.

The rescuer may note that the victim has resumed breathing with the airway opening maneuvers. Continued maintenance of an open airway may be the only rescue action required at this point.

Comment: Confirmation of breathlessness by this basic CPR step introduces the entire spectrum of airway management problems in cardiac arrest. The ACLS team leader will be responsible for

Table 3–1. ABCs: BASIC CPR SEQUENCE (ONE-PERSON)

A—Airway
A—Assess (determine unresponsiveness)
Ask for help
Appropriate positions for victim/rescuer
Airway (open: head tilt/chin lift)
B—Breathing
B—Breathing normally?
Blow in 2 breaths*
C—Circulation
C—Check for a pulse
Call the EMS system
Compress the chest†

*Take 1–1.5 seconds/ventilation.
†Compression/ventilation ratio: 15/2; compression rate = 80–100/minute.
Reassess after 4 cycles of 15 compressions and 2 ventilations.
NOTE: Adaptations for two-person CPR are: (1) two-person compression/ventilation ratio = 5/1; (2) after every 5th compression, stop for 1–1.5 seconds to allow ventilation.

all aspects of airway management throughout the resuscitation attempt. Is the absence of air movement due to an obstructed airway? What maneuver should be performed to check for an obstructed airway? If the airway is obstructed, how should it be cleared? If ventilations are needed, what ventilatory adjunct should be used? What rate and volume of ventilations are optimal? Are the ventilations effective? Many of these topics are discussed below and in Chapter 6, Airway Management.

7. Ventilate the Patient: Provide Two Rescue Breaths Over 2 to 3 Seconds. If mouth-to-mouth rescue breathing is used, the rescuer gently pinches the patient's nostrils shut with the thumb and index finger of the hand on the forehead. The rescuer takes a deep breath and places his or her open mouth around the victim's mouth so that an airtight seal is formed. A deep breath is then blown into the victim's mouth to a volume that is about twice the normal resting tidal volume. If the air entered easily, then a second deep breath is exhaled into the victim's mouth. These two breaths should be delivered in 2 to 3 seconds.

Comment: The rescuer must make several important observations at this point. First, did the air of the first breath go in? Did the chest rise? Could the rescuer hear the sound of air escaping during the passive exhalation? If air did not escape, steps must be taken to correct what may be an obstructed airway.

The rescuer must quickly repeat the head-tilt/chin-lift maneuvers and try again. If air still does not enter, consider the jaw-thrust maneuver. If still unsuccessful, then the person by definition has an obstructed airway, and the protocols for the obstructed airway, discussed later in this chapter, must be followed. The next step, closed-chest compressions, will be completely ineffective if the patient cannot be successfully ventilated.

Note AHA Standards Change:

The AHA Guidelines now recommend that the initial ventilation efforts no longer be four "stacked" breaths, delivered in rapid succession, with no exhalation between each breath. Instead, ventilations with a slower inspiratory flow rate are recommended, so that the esophageal opening pressure will not be exceeded and the chances of gastric distention, regurgitation, and aspiration are decreased.

In addition, the four stacked breaths were eliminated because the physiologic rationale behind them is now considered invalid. Cadaver studies have demonstrated that two breaths serve as well as four to increase the residual volume and open collapsed alveoli. It is also difficult physically to deliver a succession of breaths with the volumes "stair-stepping" one upon another, because exhalation of the previous breath occurs too quickly.

Teaching two slow ventilations also simplifies learning the steps of one-rescuer CPR for the layperson. The four initial ventilations (which differ from the number recommended for subsequent ventilations), and the technique of these rapid, difficult ventilations are additional details that the lay rescuer must remember. Evaluation studies have demonstrated that a sense of confusion and intimidation about "getting it just right" has led many individuals to admit that they would not attempt CPR if faced with a patient in cardiac arrest.

Circulation

8. Confirmation of Pulselessness. Once breathlessness is established, the rescuer should quickly check for a pulse at the carotid artery on the side closest to the rescuer. The pulse check should last for 5–10 seconds, because a pulse may be present, but slow irregular, or weak and rapid. The other hand is used to maintai the head-tilt position.

Comment: The rescuer has now confirmed a "full" cardia arrest—the victim is unconscious, unresponsive, breathless, and without a pulse. CPR with chest compressions and artificial ventilations is needed at once. The pulse check, which seems so simple and straightforward to hospital and emergency personnel, is difficult. Carotid pulses in the 60–80 mm HG range are notoriously difficult to detect. Failure to perform a pulse check has consistently been the most frequent error when the skills of CPR are evaluated.

9. Activate the Emergency Medical System (if not already done). If pulselessness is confirmed, the person who responded to the initial CALL FOR HELP should now be sent to activate the emergency medical system, if the arrest occurred outside the hospital, or sent to retrieve ACLS equipment and the hospital code team if the arrest occurred in the hospital.

A single rescuer faces the dilemma of whether to leave a patient who requires CPR to activate the EMS system or to stay at the patient's side and continue CPR. There are no clear limits to the maximum time that CPR can be interrupted to activate the EMS. If the patient has shown no signs of response to CPR after 1–2 cycles, we recommend that CPR should cease while the EMS system is activated. This assumes that activation of the EMS system will take no longer than 1 to 2 minutes.

10. Perform Closed-Chest Compressions. The chest should be bare if possible. Clothes should be removed quickly, down to an undergarment if necessary. The correct position for hand placement is important, to prevent complications of CPR such as liver lacerations, rib fractures, pneumo- or hemothoraces, and sternal-costal dislocation.

The rescuer feels for the lower edge of the rib cage and follows the rib edge to the notch where the ribs meet the sternum. The tip of the middle finger is placed in this notch, and the tip of the index finger falls over the lower end of the bony sternum. The heel of the other hand is then placed on the sternum, next to the index finger of the palpating hand. The fingers of this hand are kept either extended or interlaced with the fingers of the other hand throughout chest compressions. The hand used to palpate the rib edge and notch between the ribs and the sternum is now positioned over the hand on the sternum. The rescuer should be as close as possible to the side of the patient, with the shoulders directly over the patient's sternum. There should be minimal flexion of the rescuer's arms at the elbows, with most of the force of compression coming from the weight of the rescuer's upper body.

Chest compressions are initiated at a rate of 80–100/min. This rate can be achieved by counting, out loud, "one, and two, and three, and four," etc. The compressions should be smooth and steady, without bouncing, snapping, or jerking. Such undesired movements usually occur when the rescuer fails to follow the recommended compression/relaxation ratio of 50:50. Relaxation of the compression should be partially resisted by the rescuer as the hands are gradually brought up from the lowest point of the compression. The hands are not removed from contact with the chest.

Comment: One of the most consistent observations from the physiology laboratory has been the greater importance of compression *duration* relative to compression *rate*. Animal studies have shown that carotid blood flow increases with increased duration of compression. A compression duration of 60% of the compression-relaxation cycle produces a significantly higher forward carotid flow. Variations in the rate, however, in the range of 40–80 times per minute, do not appear to significantly affect carotid blood flow.

These observations underscore the importance of smooth, steady compression and relaxation without the bouncing, jerking movements so often observed on television, and at actual cardiac arrests. In practice, greater attention is often directed to maintaining the correct rate. Rescuers must concentrate less on exact 80/min chest compressions, and more on maintaining *each* compression for the required amount of time.

From the physiologic standpoint, a more relaxed rate of 40–60 compressions per minute, with prolongation of the compression duration to 60% of the cycle, may be superior and has been proposed. It is very difficult, however, to maintain that compression/relaxation ratio at such a slow rate. At the 1985 Standards Conference, the American Heart Association reviewed much of these physiologic data and concluded that, at the present time, no changes would be recommended in the method of chest compressions other than an increase in the external chest compression rate. This faster compression rate has two effects: (1) the compression/relaxation duration is optimized, and (2) a ventilatory pause is now possible to allow for a slower and more physiologic inspiratory flow rate.

COMMENT ON TWO–PERSON CPR: CHANGES IN THE VENTILATION/COMPRESSION RATIO, AND IN THE COUNTING APPROACH

A common emphasis in the teaching of basic two-person CPR has been to minimize any interruptions in the steady delivery of 60 chest compressions per minute. It was thought that chest compressions imparted momentum to the blood, and that only by continuous, uninterrupted chest compressions could this momentum be maintained.

Two problems resulted from this emphasis. First, community CPR training required complex and precise performance that wa difficult for most lay persons to achieve. Evaluation studies showec that "correct" CPR was not being performed, and that the level of skill retention declined markedly within weeks of initial training. There was some evidence that lay persons often did not attempt CPR on cardiac arrest patients they witnessed despite having completed a CPR training class. The explanation given was a fear of doing something wrong during their attempts, a fear that arose to some extent from the intimidating atmosphere that was present when they were initially taught CPR.

Second, regular chest compressions at a rate of 60/min require that ventilation volumes (recommended to be greater than 800 ml) be delivered in less than 0.5 second, during the relaxation phase of every fifth chest compression cycle. Delivery of this tidal volume in such a brief period generates tremendous pressure in both the trachea and the esophagus. This pressure is sufficiently high that it will exceed the opening pressure of the esophageal-gastric sphincter. It has been estimated that with standard two-person CPR, over 80% of each ventilation should enter the stomach, producing gastric distention and increasing the chances of regurgitation and subsequent aspiration.

In addition, recent observations about the physiology of blood flow during chest compressions have revealed that blood flow is highest for the first or second compression after a ventilation. In other words, the blood does not acquire momentum from each successive chest compression, but instead is being pumped primarily by the combination of chest compressions and the increased intrathoracic pressure that immediately follows a ventilation.

The AHA considered these observations during the 1985 Standards Conference and made the following recommendations for two-person CPR:

1. The two-rescuer technique should not be taught to the lay community. Teaching only one-rescuer CPR should result in better skill retention and possibly better performance. When a second rescuer is available at the scene, it is recommended that the second rescuer be used to activate the EMS system (if not done previously) and to perform one-rescuer CPR when the first rescuer, who initiated CPR, becomes fatigued.

2. A "ventilatory pause" should occur during the chest compressions. This pause in compressions will allow full ventilatory volumes to be delivered at slower inspiratory flow rates and lower airway pressures, thus reducing the possibility of gastric inflation and regurgitation. Adequate time (3–5 seconds) should be allowed for two full ventilations to be delivered.

3. The rate of chest compressions during two-rescuer CPR should increase to 80–100/minute. This is because the pause for ventilation decreases the total number of compressions per minute, which in turn affects the blood flow to vital organs. The faster rate will allow a total of at least 60 compressions per minute.

AIRWAY MANAGEMENT DURING BASIC CPR

Airway management is arguably the most important aspect of both basic and advanced life support. Chapter 6 presents management of the airway *performed with devices*; that is, the use of equipment, beginning with the oropharyngeal airway and the pocket face mask, and ending with the endotracheal tube. This chapter discusses management of the airway unaided by devices and performed with the *hands of the rescuer.*

Axioms of Airway Management

There are several axioms of airway management during basic CPR that must be kept always in mind:

1. Chest compressions are totally ineffective without proper ventilation.

2. An obstructed airway in a cardiac arrest patient is more likely due to the person's relaxed anatomic structures (tongue, epiglottis) than to a foreign body;

3. Always check quickly for loose dentures or an object in the mouth that may be an airway obstruction;

4. Never forget the high frequency of *secondary cardiac arrest*, which occurs when the heart has stopped beating effectively because of a lethal arrhythmia that in turn was due to a primary respiratory problem, such as a foreign body obstruction, drowning or near drowning, respiratory depression from the pharmacologic effects of drugs or from neurologic or musculoskeletal disease, and primary pulmonary disease.

5. Anybody—infant, child, or adult—who is observed at one point in time to be functioning relatively normally, and then within a short time is discovered down and unresponsive, always must be considered to have an acute airway obstruction until proved otherwise. Some examples:

   a. A small child is observed playing with small, tracheal-sized objects and then is discovered unresponsive.

   b. A small child runs about the house laughing and talking while eating an apple and suddenly turns blue and collapses.

   c. A woman hurriedly excuses herself while dining at a restaurant and is discovered a few minutes later collapsed on the floor of the women's restroom.

   d. A small child in a high chair is helped in eating finger foods by a slightly older sibling; a few minutes later the child is found slumped over and blue.

The Obstructed Airway

Much of the benefit of basic CPR training comes from its emphasis on what to do for the person who is choking from acute airway obstruction. There are several scenarios that must be learned:

1. Person in cardiac arrest who cannot be ventilated with initial two breaths

2. Person who is *choking and conscious* with

   a. incomplete obstruction (fair to good air exchange)

   b. complete obstruction (poor to no air exchange)

3. Person who is *choking and becomes unconscious*

4. Markedly obese choking victim or person in advanced stage of pregnancy

1. Person in Cardiac Arrest Who Cannot Be Ventilated with Initial Two Breaths. A rescuer may arrive at the point in basic CPR at which he or she attempts to ventilate the patient and finds that the breaths cannot be delivered. At that moment the rescuer must immediately begin the obstructed airway protocol. The rescuer should perform the following steps:

 a. Reinspect the mouth and upper airway for evidence of foreign body obstruction.

 b. Readjust the head and chin and try again; if the chest wall still does not rise with each attempted ventilation, the rescuer must assume a foreign body is present and proceed to step c, which describes a maneuver specifically developed to dislodge and expel an object that obstructs the airway.

 c. *Two manual subdiaphragmatic abdominal thrusts* (alternatively referred to as abdominal thrusts, or the Heimlich maneuver). These thrusts are performed in the following manner:

  (1) The rescuer assumes a position either astride or alongside the patient, though alongside is preferred, since the rescuer is already in that position. The heel of one hand is placed against the patient's abdomen, well below the tip of the xiphoid and in the midline, slightly above the umbilicus. The second hand is placed on top of the first.

  (2) The rescuer then presses into the patient's abdomen with two quick inward and upward thrusts.

 d. If a foreign body is not visibly expelled by the abdominal thrusts, the *finger-sweep maneuver* is performed. The rescuer turns the patient's head up and opens the mouth by lifting the tongue and lower jaw forward with the thumb and fingers; the hooked index finger of the other hand then sweeps deeply from one side of the posterior pharynx to the other.

 e. The rescuer again attempts to ventilate the lungs. If the airway remains blocked, the sequence of repositioning, abdominal thrusts, finger sweeps, and ventilation attempts must be repeated. Six to ten thrusts may be required to clear the airway. If the hypoxia persists, muscle relaxation may occur, and the previously unsuccessful attempts to relieve airway obstruction may be effective. REMEMBER: Airway obstruction must be relieved before any further steps in CPR are attempted.

2. Person Choking and Conscious. In this situation a person often demonstrates the universal sign of respiratory distress—hand clutched to throat, distressed facial expression. A distinction is made between good air exchange and poor air exchange. With good air exchange, the patient is essentially left alone; the rescuer should not interfere with the attempts of such a person to expel the foreign body by deep breaths and forceful coughing. With poor air exchange, the patient has respiratory distress, with a weak, ineffective cough, often inspiratory stridor, and little or no ability to speak. In this situation the rescuer should immediately perform the two abdominal thrusts:

a. The rescuer stands behind the patient and wraps his or her arms around the waist of the victim.

b. A fist is made with one hand and placed against the victim's epigastric area, with the thumb side toward the rescuer.

c. The free hand is placed around the fist, and two quick upward thrusts are delivered.

d. Often a foreign body is dislodged enough to be reached with the finger sweep described above.

e. This sequence must be repeated as long as the patient is distressed and remains conscious.

3. Person Choking and Becomes Unconscious. In this situation the rescuer should gently assist the victim to the floor, in the supine position, and proceed with the abdominal thrusts and finger sweeps from either astride or beside the victim.

4. Markedly Obese Choking Victim or Person in Advanced Stage of Pregnancy: The Chest Thrusts. The chest-thrust maneuver is now recommended only for the massively obese choking victim, or for a choking woman in the later months of pregnancy. If the victim is still conscious, the rescuer should:

a. Stand behind the person and encircle his or her chest.

b. Place the fist of one hand (thumb side against the chest) on the middle of the breastbone. The xiphoid process and the margins of the rib cage must be avoided.

c. Place the other hand on top of the fist and perform backward thrusts until the foreign body is expelled or the victim becomes unconscious.

d. If the victim becomes unconscious, the rescuer should place the victim on the victim's back, kneel close to the side of the victim's body, and apply chest thrusts in the same hand position that is used for external cardiac compressions.

Note AHA Standards Change:

The 1985 AHA Standards made two changes in the recommended approach to the management of the obstructed airway. First, *the four back blows are no longer recommended*. Laboratory research has suggested that back blows do not generate sufficient force to expel air from the lungs and therefore do not result in expulsion of the foreign body. Research also suggests that a force applied to the back of a patient with a foreign body lodged in the hypopharynx or in the trachea would actually be more likely to cause the object to lodge *deeper* in the trachea than to loosen the object.

The second change from previous recommendations was elimination of the chest thrust as the preferred method for relief of foreign-body airway obstruction in the adult. The Heimlich maneuver was first described in 1975. At the time of the 1979 Standards Conference, the evidence in support of the efficacy of the Heimlich maneuver was predominately anecdotal. Concern over damage to the liver, the stomach, and other abdominal organs led to recommendation of the chest thrust as the method of first choice, and the subdiaphragmatic abdominal thrust as described by Heimlich as the second choice. By the time of the 1985 Standards Conference, hard scientific evidence supporting the subdiaphragmatic abdominal thrust technique as more effective and safer than the chest thrust was still lacking. However, to improve CPR training in terms of simplifying techniques and in hopes of increasing skills retention, it was decided to select only one airway clearance technique. Because of the immense national and international publicity that the abdominal thrust, as described by Heimlich, had received, and because much of the populace was familiar, to some degree, with the Heimlich maneuver, the 1985 Standards Conference decided to choose the subdiaphragmatic abdominal thrust as the recommended maneuver.

Open-Chest Cardiac Massage

A number of articles have appeared recently with the purpose of rekindling enthusiasm for the "simple but neglected procedure" of open-chest cardiac massage. In our opinion, advocates of a dramatic increase in the frequency of open-chest CPR have erred in several respects. First, they have inappropriately generalized from physiologic data that document extremely low flow during conventional CPR to conclude that early CPR for humans will not improve survival. Second, they have accepted at first reading the conclusions of several methodologically flawed studies that have observed no benefit for bystander-initiated CPR. Third, they have uncritically accepted the conclusions of several simplistic case series published about open-chest cardiac massage in the 1950s and 1960s.

Nevertheless, appropriate indications for open-chest CPR do exist. The current absolute and relative indications for open-chest CPR are:

A. Absolute indications for open-chest CPR:
   1. Exsanguinating chest injuries
   2. Hemoperitoneum with shock
   3. Refractory cardiovascular collapse
   4. Pericardial tamponade refractory to pericardiocentesis
   5. Anatomic inability to perform closed-chest CPR (such as massive flail, pectus excavatum, scoliosis)
B. Relative indications for open-chest CPR:
   1. Severe hypothermia
   2. Refractory VF
   3. Ventricular aneurysm
   4. Severe valvular disease

5. Massive pulmonary embolism
6. Documented inadequate blood flow or oxygenation during closed chest CPR

In the near future there may emerge from responsible controlled clinical trials additional indications for open-chest cardiac massage. These might include prolonged arrest time, or failure to respond promptly to drugs, countershock, and conventional external CPR. The only randomized trial of open-chest CPR for patients in medical cardiac arrest was stopped after use in 49 patients, because no benefit was observed (Geehr, 1986).

REFERENCES

American Heart Association: Standards and guidelines for cardiopulmonary resuscitation and emergency cardiac care. JAMA 255:2905, 1986.

Babbs CF: New versus old theories of blood flow during CPR. Crit Care Med 8:191, 1980.

Bircher N, Safar P: Open-chest CPR: an old method whose time has returned. Am J Emerg Med 2:568, 1984.

Cummins RO, Eisenberg MS: Prehospital cardiopulmonary resuscitation: is it effective? JAMA 253:2408, 1985.

Cummins RO, Eisenberg MS, Hallstrom AP, et al: Survival of out-of-hospital cardiac arrest with early initiation of cardiopulmonary resuscitation. Am J Emerg Med 3:114, 1985.

Day RL, Crelin ES, DuBois AB: Choking: the Heimlich abdominal thrust vs. back blows: an approach to measurement of inertial and aerodynamic forces. Pediatrics 70:113, 1982.

Day RL: Differing opinions on the emergency treatment of choking. Pediatrics 1983;71:976, 1983.

Del Guerco LRM: A plea for open-chest CPR. Am J Emerg Med 2:565, 1984.

Eisenberg MS, Bergner L, Hallstrom A: Cardiac resuscitation in the community: importance of rapid provision and implications for program planning. JAMA 241:1905, 1979.

Geehr EC, Auerbach PS: Open-chest cardiac massage for victims of medical cardiac arrest [letter]. N Engl J Med 315:1189, 1986.

Guildner CW: Resuscitation—opening the airway: a comparative study of techniques for opening an airway obstructed by the tongue. JACEP 5:588, 1976.

Instructors Manual for Basic Life Support. Dallas, American Heart Association, 1985.

Melker R: Recommendations for ventilation during cardiopulmonary resuscitation: time for change? Crit Care Med 13:882, 1985.

Sanders AB, Ewy GA: Open-chest CPR: not yet. Am J Emerg Med 2:566, 1984.

Sanders AB, Kern KB, Ewy GA, et al: Improved resuscitation from cardiac arrest with open-chest massage. Ann Emerg Med 13:672, 1984.

4

AIRWAY MANAGEMENT

INTRODUCTION

Basic Airway Management Without Devices

Chapter 3 included airway management without adjunct devices—the use of only the rescuer's mouth and hands to provide basic life support. These approaches are vital to basic cardiopulmonary resuscitation, and for prevention of cardiac arrest in respiratory crises. Basic airway management focuses on correction of airway occlusion due to anatomic structures. The essential skills of airway management without devices are:

1. Assessment of breathlessness ("look, listen, and feel" technique)
2. Head-tilt/chin-lift technique
3. Head-tilt/jaw-thrust technique
4. Jaw-thrust technique with in-line cervical spine stabilization
5. Finger sweep
6. Chest thrust
7. Subdiaphragmatic abdominal thrust

Whenever there is loss of consciousness, the upper airway may be obstructed, although the exact mechanism of this obstruction is still disputed. Recent bronchoscopy studies suggest that the main cause of upper airway obstruction may not be the sagging tongue, as traditionally taught, but rather the epiglottis. Negative pressure can be produced in the victim's airway during inspiration. If an unconscious person is making an inspiratory effort, a negative pressure may be created in the airway. Both the epiglottis and the tongue, close to the posterior wall of the pharynx, may thus act as a valve to occlude the airway during inspiratory efforts. The basic life support maneuvers of head tilt/chin lift and the jaw-thrust technique will usually relieve upper airway obstruction, regardless of whether the tongue or the epiglottis has produced the obstruction.

These maneuvers, performed without devices, are critical for all rescuers to learn and master. If the head is in a neutral position, for example, oropharyngeal and nasopharyngeal airways will frequently fail to provide a clear airway.

Table 4–1. CORE SKILLS OF AIRWAY MANAGEMENT FOR BASIC AND ADVANCED LIFE SUPPORT PERSONNEL

1. Manual techniques of positioning and ventilation
   a. Flat on the back
   b. Chin lift/head tilt
   c. Jaw thrust/head tilt
   d. Mouth-to-mouth: expired air ventilation
2. Devices used by basic life support personnel
   a. Oral airway
   b. Pocket face mask: mouth-to-mask; expired air or with attached oxygen
   c. Nasopharyngeal airway
   d. Bag-valve-mask
   e. NOT RECOMMENDED: oxygen-powered breathing devices
3. Devices used by advanced life support personnel
   For Airway Control:
   a. Endotracheal intubation
   b. Trauma patients: orotracheal intubation with in-line stabilization
   Controversial, Generally Not Recommended:
   c. Esophageal obturator airway (EOA)
   d. Esophageal gastric-tube airway (EGTA)
   e. Digital or tactile intubation
   f. Lighted stylet intubation
   For Ventilation:
   g. Cricothyrotomy
   h. Transtracheal catheter ventilation (jet insufflation)
   For Combined Airway Control and Ventilation:
   i. Endotracheal intubation
   j. Nasotracheal intubation

Airway Management with Devices: The Personnel Approach (Table 4–1)

This chapter will review the most important devices used for airway control and for ventilation. We present a *personnel approach* because different categories of rescue personnel use different airway management devices. For better coordination of care, it is critical that all levels of personnel be familiar with the techniques used by other levels. For out-of-hospital cardiac arrest, this personnel approach parallels the sequence of application. Personnel in the emergency room must understand the proper method of head positioning for airway protection in the trauma victim, and the best way to ventilate using the bag-valve-mask unit. In turn, advanced life support personnel will often be called to employ a sequence of airway control that begins with the most basic techniques of positioning and airway control.

Basic life support personnel must thoroughly master these devices:

1. Oropharyngeal airway
2. Nasopharyngeal airway
3. Pocket face mask
4. Bag-valve-mask unit

NOT RECOMMENDED: oxygen-powered breathing devices

Advanced life support personnel must thoroughly master all of the above, plus the following devices and approaches:

5. Endotracheal intubation (including in-line)
6. Cricothyrotomy
7. Transtracheal jet insufflation

The Distinction Between Airway Control and Ventilation

Airway control means that the patient's airway is kept open and protected from occlusion either from foreign substances and objects or from anatomic structures. Once airway control is achieved, the patient must then be *ventilated*.

Ventilation can be properly assessed only by measurement of arterial blood gases. Successful ventilation means that sufficient oxygen is supplied to tissues by the blood while simultaneously carbon dioxide is eliminated. Adequate alveolar ventilation is confirmed by an arterial P_{CO_2} of 35–45 mm Hg, and an arterial P_{O_2} of 80 mm Hg or more. To achieve these ends, the patient's airway must be controlled while oxygen is moved into the patient's lungs and carbon dioxide is moved out. In emergency medical care, proper ventilation technique refers to all the approaches used to move air, usually with oxygen supplementation, into the lungs, and expired air out of the lungs.

DEVICES USED IN BASIC LIFE SUPPORT

This chapter will not give a detailed description of all devices. Instead, the commentary on each device concentrates on details of indications and proper usage.

Basic Life Support Airway Control

Oropharyngeal Airway

The oropharyngeal airway serves to hold the tongue away from the posterior wall of the pharynx. It is an important and frequently used device for airway control in unconscious patients, even if spontaneous ventilations are present.

Note, however, that the gag reflex, leading to vomiting, will be stimulated if this device is inserted into patients who are not fully comatose. It must be used only in unconscious patients who have an absent or diminished gag reflex.

If the head is *not* tilted back, the airway may still be occluded by the epiglottis and other anatomic structures of the posterior pharynx.

The tongue may be pushed backward into the posterior pharynx by the oropharyngeal airway if the latter is not inserted correctly.

The device is inserted backwards and then rotated into the

proper position. Alternatively, a tongue depressor can be used to push the tongue out of the way.

Nasopharyngeal Airway (the "Nasal Trumpet")

This device is used frequently in conscious patients, who could not otherwise tolerate the stimulation to vomit and gag from the oropharyngeal airway. Inserted through the nostrils, the device passes behind the tongue and provides a conduit for the passage of air.

The nasopharyngeal airway is particularly useful in patients with acute allergic reactions and angioedema. Also, the device can be prophylactically inserted in spontaneously ventilating patients with mild obtundation following seizures, alcohol or other drug intoxications, or cerebrovascular events.

For patient comfort, an anesthetic lubricant should be placed on sterile gauze. The nasopharyngeal airway is then drawn through the lubricant to thoroughly coat the soft rubber tube before insertion.

Basic Life Support Ventilation

Basic life support personnel have two major devices for ventilation, the pocket face mask (or pocket mask) and the bag-valve-mask unit. Evaluation studies have demonstrated that rescue personnel at the level of basic EMT can master and properly use the bag-valve-mask unit. The overwhelming majority of basic support personnel, however, will find that without proper training, regular practice and frequent field use, the bag-valve-mask becomes at best only a marginal ventilation device. These same comments are true for the emergency room and intensive care physicians—they should devote as much attention to proficiency with the pocket face mask as the bag-valve-mask device. They may well find that on those occasions during which they must ventilate a nonintubated patient, they will do as well, if not better, with the pocket mask.

Pocket Face Mask

Because of concern about disease transmission and the unpleasant and unesthetic aspects of direct oral contact with a cardiac arrest victim, emergency personnel strongly prefer the pocket face mask over mouth-to-mouth ventilation. There is no evidence, however, that the pocket face mask is more effective than direct mouth-to-mouth ventilation.

The main advantage of the pocket mask, in addition to its superior acceptability, is its oxygen insufflation nipple. With supplemental oxygen delivered at flow rates of 15 liters per minute, the pocket face mask provides an inspired oxygen concentration of about 50–80%.

For basic life support personnel, the pocket face mask is clearly superior to the bag-valve-mask unit as a ventilation device. The simplicity of the pocket face mask makes it easier to learn initially than the bag-valve-mask.

Evaluation studies have shown that many rescue personnel, including EMTs, paramedics, and physicians, have difficulty obtaining a proper seal with the bag-valve-mask. The resuscitation bags supplied with bag-valve-mask units generally supply no more than 1.0 to 1.5 liters per inflation. If any mask leakage occurs, it is difficult to deliver the recommended inflation volume of 800 cc or more. The pocket mask, in contrast, can provide up to 4 liters' of inflation volume, since the rescuer's vital capacity supplies the insufflation.

The rescuer's position for use of the pocket face mask is standing at the head of patients in bed or on stretchers, or kneeling or lying prone at the head of patients who are on the ground or the floor.

The pocket face mask should be sealed against the patient's face by *two hands*. The thumbs clamp the mask firmly to the face, while the fingers *pull the jaw upward*. As with the bag-valve-mask, the rescuer should note that as much force is applied pulling the jaw upward as is spent pushing the mask down against the skin. The mouth should remain open under the mask.

As with the bag-valve-mask, careful attention must be paid to maintenance of correct head tilt/chin lift while ventilations are provided.

Another advantage of the pocket mask is for use in trauma patients. Since the user provides maximal displacement of the mandible forward (the jaw thrust maneuver), full backward tilt of the head may not be necessary.

Only transparent pocket masks should be used, so that the rescuer can immediately detect cyanosis, vomiting, mucus, and blood. Additionally, the clouding that occurs with exhalations provides an excellent means of monitoring the patient who has returned to spontaneous respirations.

Bag-Valve-Mask Unit, with Oxygen

The major advantage of the bag-valve-mask unit over mouth-to-mouth or mouth-to-mask ventilation is its ability to deliver 100% oxygen when the bag is attached to an oxygen tank at 10 liters per minute *and* an oxygen reservoir bag is attached. Without a reservoir bag, the inhaled oxygen concentration is only 30 to 50%, and thus the bag-valve-mask loses any ventilation advantages over the pocket face mask used with O_2.

Several studies, however, have documented the strong preference that emergency personnel have for the bag-valve-mask over the pocket face mask. This appears to be partly due to the

Table 4–2. THE "FATS" TECHNIQUE (FACE AND THIGH SQUEEZE) FOR BAG-VALVE-MASK VENTILATION*

1. The patient should be flat on his or her back. The rescuer is positioned at the patient's head, kneeling.
2. Tilt the patient's head backward, and maintain this backward tilt by pressure from the thighs of the rescuer.
3. Place the mask over the patient's mouth and nose, pressing firmly with the palm of the hand. The fingers grip the edge of the mandible and pull *upward*. In effect, the mask is clamped firmly to the face by a gripping effect of the fingers pulling the mandible upward, and the palm pushing the mask downward.
4. The resuscitation bag is firmly squeezed between the other hand and the thigh. Attempt to completely empty the bag. Attempts to squeeze the bag with the hand alone seldom meet with success.
5. Watch for the chest to rise; listen for the sound of escaping air that indicates a poor mask-to-face seal.
6. Abruptly release the bag for exhalation. A quick bag release is necessary for proper valve function.

*Recommended for field resuscitation by basic life support personnel.

difference in aesthetics between the two devices, some unjustified concern over disease transmission, and the sense of greater professional status associated with the use of the bag-valve-mask.

Given that basic life support personnel have a strong preference for the bag-valve-mask device, it is critically important that the task of ventilating with the bag-valve-mask be completed mastered, and such mastery documented.

Table 4–2 presents a recommended technique for ventilation with the bag-valve-mask unit that differs from the standard description given in most life support textbooks. The advantages of this technique are that it reduces operator problems in establishing and maintaining a seal and it provides full compression of the resuscitation bag.

Because use of the bag-valve-mask unit will often cause the mouth to close under the mask, an oropharyngeal tube should be used simultaneously, to help maintain airway patency and to overcome nasal obstruction.

The two-rescuer technique, in which one rescuer keeps the airway open and maintains a tight seal while the second rescuer squeezes the bag with both hands, frequently solves problems by achieving a tight seal between the mask and the face of the victim.

Oxygen Supplementation
Nasal Cannula

The nasal cannula can deliver oxygen concentrations of 25–40% when the flow rate is 6 liters per minute. It should be used only on spontanenously breathing patients.

Plastic Face Mask

The plastic face mask can deliver oxygen concentrations of 50–60% when the flow rate is 10 liters per minute.

Venturi Mask

The concentrations of O_2 available through various Venturi masks are 24% and 28% (when flow is 4 L/min), and 35% and 40% (when flow is 8 L/min).

The Venturi mask provides good control of the inspired O_2 and thus is most suitable for patients with chronic hypercarbia from chronic pulmonary disease.

Often there is concern that a patient with chronic lung disease may have chronic hypoxia-driven respirations. Consequently, administration of high levels of oxygen may produce respiratory depression and hypercarbia. Administration of 24% or 28% O_2 through a Venturi mask may significantly relieve hypoxemia but will not cause respiratory depression in a patient with chronic carbon dioxide retention. If no signs of respiratory depression are observed, the next highest concentration of O_2 through the Venturi mask can be used.

Controversial Devices for Basic Life Support Airway Management: Manually Triggered Oxygen-Powered Breathing Devices

Basic life support personnel should *not* use oxygen-powered breathing devices, despite the fact that some emergency medical systems have adopted them. In basic life support, there are no advantages to oxygen-powered devices over the pocket face mask or the bag-valve-mask. In addition, there is little evidence that such devices have a role to play in advanced cardiac life support. Together with this lack of significant advantages, the following serious disadvantages render these devices unacceptable:

1. These pressure-cycled devices cannot be used during external chest compression, because chest compressions prematurely terminate the inflation cycle, leading to inadequate ventilation.

2. The high pressures generated by these devices cause gastric insufflation, regurgitation, lung rupture, and tension pneumothorax.

3. The devices are heavy, clumsy, dependent on compressed gas, and can interfere with other, more significant activities during resuscitation attempts.

4. Extensive training, practice, and retraining are required for correct use.

5. Finally, in comparison with the use of the pocket face mask or the bag-valve-mask, the rescuer loses the feel of the compliance or ease of filling of the lungs, and the early detection of partial obstruction from the accumulation of secretions in the airway.

DEVICES USED IN ADVANCED LIFE SUPPORT

The authors of this book approach the problem of airway management by advanced life support personnel with several biases. These biases, based upon experience with a sophisticated prehospital care system and critical reading of published studies, are as follows:

1. Endotracheal intubation is the emergency airway of choice, the definitive method, the gold standard.

2. The trachea should be intubated by trained personnel as soon as practical during the course of a resuscitation.

3. However, as noted in the chapters on management of cardiac arrests, rhythm assessment and defibrillation (if the rhythm is ventricular fibrillation) should precede endotracheal intubation for patients in cardiac arrest.

4. In addition, the airway control and ventilation techniques discussed under the basic life support method, should precede attempts at tracheal intubation.

5. Advanced life support personnel should be trained and highly skilled in the use of pharmacologic adjuncts to intubation, such as succinylcholine. There should be no hesitancy to use such agents early.

6. The esophageal obturator airway and the esophageal gastric-tube airway continue to be listed as alternative approaches to emergency airway management in the standards and guidelines of the American Heart Association. The inclusion of these devices was done amid considerable controversy. In our opinion, however, these are unproved devices whose safety is highly questionable. They are completely unacceptable as alternatives to endotracheal intubation. Other than protection of the airway from regurgitated stomach contents, they have no advantages over the pocket face mask and the bag-valve-mask.

7. Given these biases, the optimal sequence that emerges for immediate airway management of a patient in cardiac arrest is:
   a. Proper positioning
   b. Oropharyngeal airway
   c. Mouth-to–pocket face mask ventilation, or bag-valve-mask
   d. Endotracheal intubation

It is of note that this is the approach to airway management used in the four emergency medical systems that have the highest published rates of resuscitation success in the United States. Adjunct devices such as mechanical CPR compressors, oxygen-powered breathing devices, and esophageal obturator airways have been studiously avoided in these systems, and yet their resuscitation rates remain consistently the nation's highest.

Advanced Life Support Airway Control

Tracheal intubation may be accomplished from a variety of approaches, both nonsurgical and surgical. For the cardiac arrest patient, this book follows the approach recommended by the American Heart Association: orotracheal intubation for definitive airway control and ventilation; and transtracheal ventilation and cricothyrotomy for ventilation of patients with obstructed airways. (As noted above, we deviate from the AHA recommendations in that we consider the EOA and the EGTA unproved and unacceptable devices.)

Current recommendations for the airway management of patients with multiple injuries, including obvious or possible cervical spine, neck, and facial injuries, is highly controversial. Advanced Trauma Life Support Classes, sponsored by the Committee on Trauma of the American College of Surgeons, and Prehospital Trauma Life Support Classes, developed by the National Association of EMTs, (and also sponsored by the Committee on Trauma of the American College of Surgeons) currently teach the technique of nasotracheal intubation with in-line stabilization. The rationale for the adoption of this technique is unclear. Numerous published studies report a high complication rate when blind nasotracheal intubation is attempted in the prehospital setting, and its use by prehospital personnel is vigorously opposed by many airway management experts. Only one study of blind nasotracheal intubation, compared with succinylcholine-assisted orotracheal intubation, has appeared (Dronen et al, 1986). In 41 obtunded drug-overdose patients, the authors observed a marked superiority of orotracheal intubation in terms of mean time to intubate, number of attempts, and associated complications.

Endotracheal Intubation

Endotracheal intubation is the quickest, simplest, and most effective method for providing ventilation and protecting the airway. It also provides an alternative route for administration of drugs such as epinephrine, lidocaine, and atropine. Ventilation and oxygenation should be provided initially by the methods discussed earlier, and tracheal intubation should be attempted as soon as possible during a resuscitation. Ventilation must not be interrupted unnecessarily or for greater than 30 seconds during attempts at intubation.

Equipment and Supplies:
1. Bag-valve-mask device with oxygen source
2. Laryngoscope with curved and straight blades (be sure that light works)
3. Endotracheal tubes of different sizes
4. Stylet (optional)
5. Suction device
6. Syringe, 10 ml
7. Sterile water-soluble lubricant
8. Adhesive tape
NOTE: Assemble all equipment and ascertain proper function before attempting to intubate.

Procedure:

1. Select the proper size tube and inflate the balloon with 5 ml of air to be sure the balloon is intact.

2. Lubricate the tube generously.

3. (Optional) Insert the stylet until the tip is approximately 1 cm proximal to the end of the endotracheal tube; then bend the stylet and tube into a crescent shape.

4. Ventilate the patient with bag-valve-mask plus 100% oxygen for 1–2 minutes. Repeat this step if any subsequent steps require more than 30 seconds to perform.

5. With the patient's head tilted backward, open the patient's mouth with the right hand. (NOTE: In patients under 1 month of age, the head should be in a neutral position.) Remove dentures and suction any secretion or vomitus.

6. Hold the laryngoscope in the left hand and insert the blade to the right of the tongue, pushing the tongue to the left while advancing the blade to the hypopharynx.

   a. *Curved blade*—the blade is inserted into the hypopharynx so that the epiglottis is still visible and is lifted with lifting of the hypopharynx.

   b. *Straight blade*—the blade is inserted below the epiglottis and actually lifts the epiglottis to expose the vocal cords.

7. Lift the laryngoscope upward and forward in one smooth motion without pivoting the blade. The vocal cord should now be visible. If an assistant is available, cricoid cartilage pressure applied with the thumb and index finger to the anterolateral aspect of the cartilage may help bring the larynx into view and prevent aspiration.

8. While visualizing the vocal cords, pass the tube along the side of the laryngoscope blade into the trachea until the balloon is just past the vocal cords.

9. Withdraw the laryngoscope and the stylet, if used.

10. Connect the bag-valve-mask and ventilate with 100% oxygen.

11. Check immediately for correct placement of the tube by listening with a stethoscope for airflow over both lung fields and the stomach. If airflow is heard in the stomach instead of the lung fields, the esophagus was intubated. Remove the tube and ventilate the patient with bag-valve-mask, then try again to intubate. If breath sounds over each side of the chest are unequal, the tube is probably inserted too far and is in the right main stem bronchus. Withdraw the tube 1–2 cm and listen again. When breath sounds are equal on both sides of the chest, inflate the endotracheal cuff with air until no air leak around the tube can be heard.

12. An oral airway may be inserted to prevent the patient from biting the tube.

13. Tape the tube securely into place by wrapping one end of the adhesive tape around the tube where it emerges from the

mouth. Extend the tape to the cheek and around the back of the neck to the other cheek. Split the end of the tape and tape the upper half to the upper lip and wrap the lower half around the tube.

14. Obtain a portable chest x-ray immediately to ascertain correct tube placement.

15. Obtain serial arterial blood gas measurements to assess adequacy of ventilation.

Advanced Life Support Ventilation

Endotracheal intubation, discussed above, provides not only definitive airway control but also definitive ventilation. There are, however, two approaches that can best be characterized as mainly ventilation adjuncts—*transtracheal catheter insufflation* and *cricothyrotomy*. The American Heart Association recommends these two approaches (as opposed to nasotracheal intubation) as advanced life support skills for the ventilation of patients with airway obstruction unmanageable with any of the previously described methods.

Transtracheal Catheter Insufflation

Of the surgical and semisurgical procedures aimed toward relieving the obstructed airway, transtracheal catheter insufflation, or jet insufflation, has the least number of complications. Rescue personnel should move at once to transtracheal catheter insufflation when nonsurgical airway management approaches have failed, or when prolonged apnea periods occur during nonsurgical airway management attempts.

In this technique, a 14-gauge plastic intravenous catheter is inserted through the cricothyroid membrane. A hand-operated release valve and intravenous extension tubing connects the catheter to a wall oxygen outlet. Oxygen, at 50 psi, is insufflated into the trachea until the lungs are visibly inflated. When the valve is released, exhalation occurs passively.

The problem with transtracheal catheter insufflation is that its major indication is airway obstruction, and yet when there is complete airway obstruction there is no way for the insufflated air to be exhaled. In this situation, a second large needle should be passed through the cricothyroid membrane to permit exhalation.

In some cases of incomplete airway obstruction, a retrograde air leak as well as exhalations will occur. This may help to expel oropharyngeal secretions.

Another advantage of transtracheal catheter insufflation is that chest compressions can be continued during the procedure. Tracheal intubation or tracheostomy can then follow in a somewhat less hectic manner.

Cricothyrotomy

Cricothyrotomy will almost always be preceded by efforts to use transtracheal catheter insufflation. An exception is the multiply-injured patient in cardiac arrest. In this situation rescue personnel should move at once to perform a cricothyrotomy.

Equipment and Supplies: Cricothyrotomy can be performed in the emergency situation with just a pocket knife. However, if possible, the following should be available, preferably in prester-ilized kits.

1. Cap, gown, mask, and gloves to maintain sterility
2. Material for sterilizing the skin
3. Sterile drapes and 4 × 4 inch gauze sponges
4. No. 11 scalpel blade with handle
5. Mosquito or Kelly clamps
6. Low-pressure endotracheal tubes or cuffed tracheostomy tubes of various sizes
7. Syringe, 10-ml
8. Bag-valve-mask with oxygen source
9. Adhesive tape
10. (If patient is conscious), lidocaine, 1%, and syringe, 5-ml, with a 25-gauge needle.

Procedure:

1. Place the patient in a supine position with the head tilted backward.
2. If time permits, sterilize a wide area of the skin of the neck and observe sterile technique by donning mask, cap, gloves, and gown.
3. Locate the cricothyroid membrane. It is the depression just below or caudal to the thyroid cartilage (Adam's apple).
4. If time permits and the patient is conscious, infiltrate the skin over the cricothyroid membrane with 1% lidocaine.
5. With the No. 11 scalpel blade or any sharp instrument (e.g., pen knife), make a transverse incision through the skin over the membrane and then puncture the membrane in the midline.
6. If available, use a mosquito or Kelly clamp to bluntly enlarge the incision. Otherwise, an adequate airway can be made just by turning the knife blade 90° from the line of incision.
7. If endotracheal or tracheostomy tubes are being used, check first to make sure the cuff is intact by inflating it with air. Insert the tube into the trachea, directing the end of the tube caudally. If endotracheal or tracheostomy tubes are not available, any thin-walled hollow instrument may be used. An example is the bottom half of a ballpoint pen that can be unscrewed.
8. Direct ventilation through the tube can be given by mouth or, if available, by bag-valve-mask unit with 100% oxygen.
9. Check for movement of the chest wall and for equal breath sounds bilaterally.

10. Cut a 4 × 4 inch gauze sponge halfway down the middle and place it over the incision and around the tube. Do not suture the incision site or bandage tightly, since subcutaneous emphysema may develop.

11. Tape or tie the tube securely into place. Be sure not to tape or tie too tightly, as this will cause venous congestion.

12. If possible, obtain a portable chest x-ray to check tube position.

MECHANICAL VENTILATION

Mechanical ventilation is an adjunct to manual ventilation with a bag-valve system. During the acute situation—either a cardiac arrest or an unstable patient—manual ventilation should be used, since the patient's pulmonary status and acid-base balance are in flux and need to be continually adjusted. Once the patient's condition stabilizes and if assisted ventilation is still necessary, the patient can be placed on a ventilator for mechanical ventilation. The following discussion briefly summarizes the ventilator settings that must be determined for optimal patient management.

Types of Ventilators

Volume-Cycled. Tidal volume and frequency are set, and pressure and I:E (inspiratory/expiratory) ratio are secondarily determined. Inspiratory phase ceases when a preset tidal volume is delivered. As lung compliance decreases, the pressure needed to deliver the tidal volume will increase. However, when the patient's lung becomes stiffer than the ventilator tubing, tidal volume may decrease as more gas goes to expansion of the tubing. This decrease in tidal volume is usually significant only in neonates and young children.

Time-Cycled. The inspiratory and expiratory time are set and tidal volume, pressure, I:E ratio, and frequency are secondarily determined. A fairly constant tidal volume is delivered regardless of changes in lung compliance. Time-cycled ventilators require more operator expertise than the other types of ventilators.

Pressure-Cycled. Pressure and frequency are set, the tidal volume and I:E ratio are secondarily determined. Inspiratory phase ceases when a preset pressure limit is reached. Tidal volume varies directly with the patient's lung compliance. Because of the potential for hypoventilation when lung compliance decreases and the fact that FIO_2 cannot be precisely set, pressure-cycled ventilators have fallen out of favor.

Ventilator Settings

Only the basic settings necessary for routine use will be discussed. More sophisticated setups should be used in consultation with a certified respiratory therapist or pulmonologist.

NOTE: Arterial blood gas measurements should be obtained 15 minutes after initiation of mechanical ventilation or after any changes in ventilator settings.

1. Tidal Volume: *Adults*: 10–15 ml/kg; *infants*: 8–12 ml/kg.

2. Frequency: *Adults*: 10–14 breaths/min for achieving normal P_{CO_2}; *infants*: 25–30 breaths/min (up to 60 for severe hyaline membrane disease).

3. Inspired Oxygen Concentration (FIo_2): 50% to 100% initially. Use the lowest FIo_2 needed to maintain oxygen-hemoglobin saturation at greater than or equal to 90%. This usually corresponds to arterial Po_2 greater than 60 mm Hg. Any shift of the hemoglobin-oxygen dissociation curve to the right (acidemia, hypercarbia, fever, hemoglobinopathies, toxins) will require a higher arterial Po_2 to maintain 90% saturation.

Pulmonary oxygen toxicity can develop within 30 hours at an FIo_2 of 1.00 and within 48 hours at 0.70. FIo_2 of 0.40 is well tolerated for over 30 days. In neonates, retrolental fibroplasia and bronchopulmonary dysplasia can develop. The time course and dose relationship is not well established.

4. Peak Pressure: *For pressure-cycled ventilator*: 20–25 cm H_2O in patients with normal lungs; 30–50 cm H_2O in patients with respiratory failure; >60 cm H_2O is associated with a high incidence of barotrauma. *For volume- or time-cycled ventilators*: set limit at 10 cm H_2O above observed initial peak pressure. If alarm sounds, the cause for increasing pressure must be sought; most frequently this will be patient override, pneumothorax, kinking of the endotracheal tube, incorrect placement of the tube, or obstruction of the tube or major airway.

5. Ventilator Mode:

   a. *Controlled ventilation*—ventilation delivered only at the preset rate. Used for patients without adequate respiratory drive or for deliberate hyperventilation.

   b. *Assist control*—the minimum ventilation rate is preset. If the patient generates a sufficient inspiratory effort, the machine will be triggered to deliver an extra breath at the preset tidal volume. This mode is usually preferred in the conscious patient.

6. Inspiratory Flow Rate: *Adults*: 40–50 L/min; *Infants*: 8–15 L/min.

7. I:E Ratio: 1:2 to 1:3, in patients with COPD or asthma; 1:4 may be needed for complete exhalation.

8. Positive End-Expiratory Pressure (PEEP): If needed, start at 5 cm H_2O and increase by 3–5 cm H_2O every 15 min as necessary. Monitor BP, P, ABG, lung compliance, and cardiac output.

9. Continuous Positive Airway Pressure (CPAP) (usually used in infants with hyaline membrane disease): 2–8 cm H_2O; if not adequate, mechanical ventilation is needed.

10. Inspired Air: should be warmed and humidified in patients who are intubated. This is also an adjunct to core rewarming of hypothermic patients.

11. Nebulizer Therapy: can be administered via mechanical ventilators in the intubated patient.

Management

In the conscious patient, sedation may be necessary to avoid anxiety, bucking the ventilator, or breathing out of phase. We recommend either Morphine, 2–4 mg IV every 5–30 min, titrating to effect, or diazepam, 2.5–5.0 mg IV up to 1 mg/kg, every 5–10 min, titrating to effect.

When sedation alone is ineffective or hypotension develops, a paralyzing agent may be added. Pancuronium, 0.02–0.06 mg/kg IV, may be given every 1–2 hours as needed.

NOTE: Although patients may appear to be asleep or unconscious, they should be treated as fully awake. Any procedures should be explained to the patient and reassurances given. Bedside discussions should be avoided.

All potential complications should be sought on a routine basis. The patient's pulmonary and hemodynamic parameters must be monitored frequently (BP, P, RR, ABGs, cardiac output, lung compliance). A cause must be determined for any increase in O_2 consumption or CO_2 production, agitation, hypotension, or change in peak pressure or tidal volume. Only after complications or malfunctions are excluded should ventilator settings be readjusted or the patient sedated.

REFERENCES

Auerback PS, Geehr EC: Inadequate oxygenation and ventilation using the esophageal gastric tube airway in the prehospital setting. JAMA *250*:3067, 1983.

Clinton JE, Ruiz E: Emergency Airway management procedures. In Roberts JR, Hedges JR (eds): Clinical Procedures in Emergency Medicine. Philadelphia, WB Saunders, 1985.

Cummins RO, Austin D, Graves JR, et al: The ventilation skills of emergency medical technicians: a teaching challenge for emergency medicine. Ann Emerg Med *15*:1187, 1986.

Dronen SC, Merigan K, Hedges J, et al: A comparison of blind nasotracheal and succinylcholine-assisted intubation in the poisoned patient. Ann Emerg Med *15*:13(A), 1986.

Melker RJ, Banner MJ: Ventilation during CPR: two-rescuer standards reappraised. Ann Emerg Med *14*:403, 1985.

Montgomery WH: Ventilation during cardiopulmonary resuscitation. In Harwood AL (ed): Cardiopulmonary Resuscitation. Baltimore, Williams & Wilkins, 1982.

Pepe PE, Copass MK, Joyce TH: Prehospital endotracheal intubation: rationale for training emergency medical personnel. Ann Emerg Med *14*:1085, 1985.

Safar P: Cardiopulmonary cerebral resuscitation: basic and advanced life support. In

Schwartz GR, Safar P, Stone JH, et al (eds): Principles and Practice of Emergency Medicine, 2nd ed. Philadelphia, WB Saunders, 1986.

Smith JP, Bodai BI, Seifkin A, et al: The esophageal obturator airway: a review. JAMA 250:1081, 1983.

White RD, Goldberg AH, Montgomery WH: Adjuncts for airway control and ventilation. In McIntyre KM, Lewis AJ (eds): Textbook of Advanced Cardiac Life Support. Dallas, American Heart Association, 1981, pp. IV1–10.

5

CENTRAL VENOUS LINES

Reliable intravenous access must be secured as soon as possible after establishing BCLS and delivering initial defibrillation to those patients in ventricular fibrillation. Preferably at least two intravenous sites with catheter size 18 gauge or greater should be available. If tracheal intubation is established before intravenous access, endotracheal administration of epinephrine, lidocaine, and atropine can also be effective.

An antecubital vein is the preferred initial site of cannulation, since at this site it can be performed easily, with few complications, and without interrupting CPR. A central line can often be established by passing a long catheter through an antecubital vein. More distal peripheral sites such as the wrist, hand, or leg should be used only as a last resort, since blood flow to these areas is low during cardiac arrest and thus drugs administered at these sites will take significantly longer to reach the heart.

The *advantages* of a central line over peripheral sites are as follows:

1. It obviates the need for intracardiac administration of drugs.

2. Administered drugs are delivered rapidly and at high concentrations to the heart.

3. Central veins are more rapidly and easily cannulated, since anatomic variation is minimal and vasoconstriction is less significant.

The *disadvantages* of a central line are:

1. Its insertion during cardiac arrest should be done only by skilled or experienced personnel.

2. CPR must be interrupted (unless a central line is already in place) for jugular and subclavian vein cannulation.

3. It is associated with a greater risk of complications, such as pneumothorax, hematoma formation, and air embolism.

4. It is a relative contraindication to thrombolytic therapy, and a missed attempt is a strong contraindication.

INTERNAL JUGULAR CANNULATION

The internal jugular site is associated with a lower risk of complication than the subclavian site and, in the intubated patient, requires minimal interruption of CPR. However, the vein is more difficult to find than the subclavian vein, and injury to the carotid artery can occur. Also, when inserted, the internal jugular catheter is more difficult to anchor securely.

Equipment and Supplies:
1. Material for skin sterilization and sterile technique
2. Intravenous fluid and tubing, assembled and flushed
3. Drapes and gauze sponges
4. Syringe, 3–5 ml, with 22-gauge, 2½-inch needle
5. Central venous catheter (at least 12 cm long) with introducing needle
6. Needle holder, scissors, and skin suture (size 4-0 or larger) on a cutting needle to anchor the line
7. Tape and topical antibacterial ointment
8. For skin anesthesia in conscious patients, 1% lidocaine and 10-ml syringe with a 25-gauge needle

Procedure:
1. Place the patient in the Trendelenburg (head-down) position, if possible, and turn the head away from the side of insertion.
2. Sterilize a large area of skin around the insertion site, and observe sterile technique.
3. The operator should stand at the patient's head on the side of the insertion site.
4. Use the syringe with the 22-gauge 2½-inch needle as a probe to find the internal jugular vein. Insert the needle, at a 30° angle to the skin, at the apex of the triangle formed by the two heads of the sternocleidomastoid muscle and the clavicle (Fig. 5–1). Advance the needle toward the ipsilateral nipple while maintaining constant pull on the plunger of the syringe. If the vein is not entered, withdraw the needle until the tip is just beneath the skin, and reposition the needle, usually medially, being careful to avoid the carotid artery. Once the vein is entered (dark blood enters the syringe), note the position and angle of the needle and withdraw the probe.
NOTE: In the conscious patient, the probe syringe can be filled with 1% lidocaine and the path of the needle anesthetized. Always aspirate before injecting, to avoid accidental intravenous injection.
5. Attach the syringe to the introducing needle of the central catheter and follow the path of the probe needle. Be sure to aspirate continuously, so as not to pass through the vein inadvertently. When blood flows into the syringe, rotate the needle 360° while aspirating to make sure that the needle tip is completely inside the vein. Disconnect the syringe and immediately occlude the hub of the needle with the thumb, to prevent air from entering.
6. Insert the central venous catheter and check that the catheter is in the vein by lowering the intravenous bag and making sure there is good blood return in the catheter.
7. *Never withdraw the catheter by itself once it is in the needle; it can be sheared off.* Remove the needle from the vein by withdrawing the catheter and needle as a single unit.
8. Place a skin suture and anchor the catheter in place. Secure

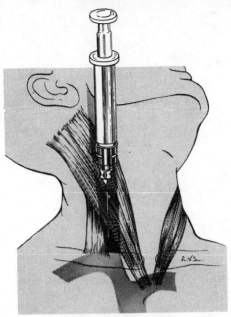

Figure 5–1. Internal jugular vein catheterization—anterior approach. (From Dunphy JE, Way LW (eds): Current Surgical Diagnosis and Treatment, 5th ed. Los Altos, CA, Lange, 1981. Reprinted with permission.)

further with tape, and dress the insertion site with antibacterial ointment and gauze.

9. Tighten and tape all connections.

10. Take the patient out of the Trendelenburg position and obtain a portable chest x-ray immediately, to ascertain the position of the catheter and check for the presence of pneumothorax.

SUBCLAVIAN VEIN CANNULATION

Subclavian vein catheterization can be performed rapidly by experienced personnel. Because it can be anchored securely, a subclavian line can be left in place for prolonged periods of time if proper antiseptic technique was used during insertion and maintenance. In addition, it provides ready access for transvenous pacemaker insertion. However, subclavian cannulation is associated with a high risk of complications, such as pneumothorax, hemothorax, and hematoma formation. Chest compressions must be discontinued during insertion of a subclavian line.

Equipment and Supplies: Same as for internal jugular vein cannulation.

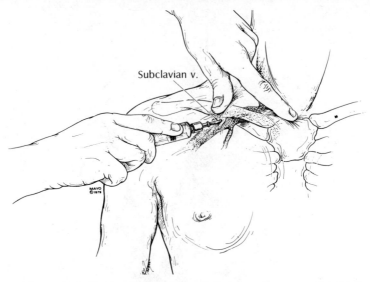

Subclavian v.

Figure 5–2. Hand position during subclavian venipuncture. (Modified from Linos D, Mucha P, von Heerden J: Subclavian vein: a golden route. Mayo Clin Proc 55:318, 1980. Used with permission.)

Procedure:

1. Place the patient in the Trendelenburg (head-down) position and hyperextend the shoulders by placing a rolled towel between the patient's scapulas. Turn the patient's head away from the side of insertion.

2. Sterilize a wide area of skin around the insertion site and observe sterile technique.

3. While standing beside and facing the patient, use the index finger to locate the costoclavicular ligament along the inferior border of the clavicle, approximately one-third the length of the clavicle from the suprasternal notch.

4. Connect a 3-ml syringe to the catheter insertion needle. Place the thumb on the clavicle over the costoclavicular ligament and the index finger of the same hand in the suprasternal notch. Insert the needle with the bevel up through the skin just below the thumb at a 10–20° angle to the skin along an imaginary line defined by the thumb and index finger (Fig. 5–2). In the conscious patient, a probe may be used to anesthetize the path of insertion.

5. When the needle touches the clavicle, decrease the angle until the syringe is parallel to the skin. Slowly move the needle inferiorly along the clavicle by repeatedly tapping the clavicle. When the inferior surface of the clavicle is reached, pull back on the plunger of the syringe to maintain a vacuum, and advance the needle parallel to the skin along the aforementioned imaginary line.

6. When blood flows into the syringe, the vein has been entered.

Rotate the needle until the bevel faces the patient's feet. Be sure blood still flows freely. Remove the syringe and immediately occlude the hub of the needle to prevent aspiration of air.

7. Insert the catheter into the vein while holding the needle in place. *Never withdraw the catheter once it is inserted into the needle or it may be sheared off and embolized.* Withdraw the catheter and needle as a single unit to remove the needle from the vein.

8. Check that the catheter is in the vein by lowering the intravenous bag and observing for backflow of blood. If the catheter is not in position, withdraw the needle and catheter as a unit and try again. Flush the insertion needle to be sure the lumen is patent.

9. Anchor the catheter to the chest by tying a skin suture, looping the suture around the catheter several times, and tying it again. Secure further with tape. Apply antibiotic ointment and dress the site.

10. Tighten and tape all connections.

11. Take the patient out of the Trendelenburg position. Immediately obtain a portable chest x-ray to ascertain correct position of the catheter and check for the presence of pneumothorax.

NOTE: Central catheters that are advanced too far into the atrium or right ventricle can cause arrhythmias.

FEMORAL VEIN CANNULATION

Femoral vein catheterization can usually be performed quickly and easily without interrupting CPR. Complications are minimal if the line is removed after the urgency is over. However, for it to be as effective as the other central lines, the catheter must be long enough to be passed above the diaphragm.

Equipment and Supplies: Same as for internal jugular vein cannulation.

Procedure:
1. Place the patient supine with the leg externally rotated.
2. Sterilize the groin area and drape. Observe sterile technique.
3. Locate the femoral vein (see Fig. 5–3). The femoral vein lies approximately at the medial third of the distance from the pubic tubercle to the anterior iliac crest. In patients with a palpable pulse, the femoral vein is 1–2 cm medial to the femoral artery.
4. Connect the syringe to the catheter insertion needle and insert the needle at a 45° angle through the skin above the femoral vein. Anesthetize the site of insertion if the patient is conscious. Pull back the plunger of the syringe as the needle is advanced. When dark blood enters the syringe, the femoral vein has been entered. Rotate the needle 360° while aspirating to be sure the tip is completely in the lumen of the vein.

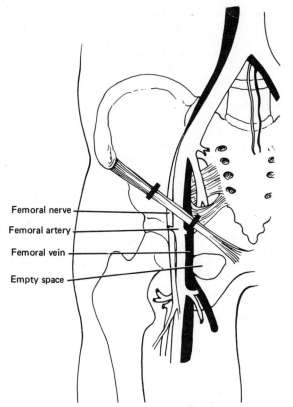

Femoral nerve

Femoral artery

Femoral vein

Empty space

Figure 5–3. Anatomic relationships of the femoral vein at the inguinal ligament. (From Mills J, Ho M, Salber P, Trunky D: Current Emergency Diagnosis and Treatment, 2nd ed. Los Altos, CA, Lange, 1985. Reprinted with permission.)

5. Pass the catheter through the needle and into the vein. Lower the intravenous bag to confirm catheter placement by checking for backflow of blood into the tubing.

6. Remove the needle from the vein by withdrawing the catheter and needle as a single unit. *Do not withdraw the catheter by itself, since it can be sheared off by the needle.*

7. Anchor the catheter with a skin suture and tape securely. Apply antibacterial ointment and dress the site.

8. Obtain a portable chest x-ray to confirm correct position of the catheter.

9. If bright red blood is aspirated into the syringe, the femoral artery may have been entered. Remove the needle and apply direct pressure for 5–10 minutes. Try again on the opposite side or the same side.

10. Once the femoral vein is catheterized, do not attempt to obtain arterial blood for blood gas measurement on the side of the catheterization.

VENOUS CUTDOWN

Venous cutdown is performed less often now, since internal jugular, subclavian, and femoral vein catheterizations have become more popular. However, it is still preferred in the severely hypovolemic patient (e.g., with severe trauma or traumatic arrest), in whom the central veins may be collapsed and rapid volume infusion through large-bore cannulas are needed. In severely hypovolemic infants and small children, saphenous vein cutdown may be the most rapid method of establishing intravenous access. Also, in patients without peripheral sites who have bleeding disorders or are anticoagulated, and who need a central line, venous cutdown allows for better hemostasis than the other methods of central venous catheterization.

On the other hand, venous cutdown is more invasive and may cause excessive delay in establishing venous access, especially when the operator is not skilled. A detailed knowledge of the course of the vein to be used and of the anatomy at the site of the cutdown is essential to success and minimizing damage to surrounding structures. Venous cutdown is contraindicated if the vein is injured proximal to the proposed cutdown site.

Equipment and Supplies:
1. Material for skin sterilization and sterile technique
2. Intravenous fluid and tubing with blood administration setup, assembled and flushed
3. Drapes and gauze sponges
4. 4-0 silk ties (2)
5. Tourniquet
6. For skin anesthesia in conscious patients, 1% lidocaine and a 10-ml syringe with a 25-gauge 1½-inch needle
7. 4-0 nylon or polypropylene suture on cutting needle
8. Needle holder
9. No. 11 and No. 15 scalpel blades mounted on holders
10. Curved Kelly clamp
11. Mosquito clamp
12. Tissue dissection scissors and suture scissors
13. Self-retaining retractor
14. Forceps
15. Catheters—5F or 10F pediatric feeding tubes or IV tubing
16. Armboard
17. Tape, antibacterial ointment, and rolled gauze bandage

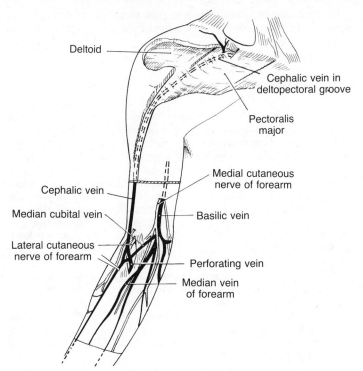

Figure 5–4. The veins of the upper limb. (From Roberts RJ, Hedges JR: Clinical Procedures in Emergency Medicine. Philadelphia, W.B. Saunders, 1985, Reprinted with permission.)

Procedure:

1. Position patient and tape limb securely to armboard as follows: for antecubital fossa cutdown—patient supine with arm extended and palm up; for saphenous cutdown—patient supine with foot externally rotated to maximally expose the medial malleolus.

2. Sterilize a wide area of skin at the cutdown site (see Figs. 5–4 and 5–5).

3. Apply the tourniquet.

4. Drape the limb and observe sterile technique.

5. Cut the catheter to the desired length by measuring, and fill with intravenous fluid. NOTE: Cut at an angle to create a bevel and trim off sharp tip.

6. In the conscious patient, infiltrate the incision site with lidocaine.

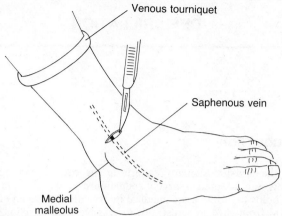

Figure 5–5. A skin incision is made perpendicular to the course of the vein. (From Roberts RJ, Hedges JR: Clinical Procedures in Emergency Medicine. Philadelphia, W.B. Saunders, 1985. Reprinted with permission.)

7. With a No. 15 scalpel, make a transverse incision perpendicular to the course of the vein to be cannulated, extending down to subcutaneous tissue and wide enough for adequate exposure.

8. Use the curved Kelly clamp to bluntly dissect and isolate the vein. The self-retaining retractor can be used for field exposure.

9. After the vein is isolated and mobilized, place an open Kelly clamp under the vein for support.

10. Two silk ties are passed under the vein with forceps and separated, one proximal and one distal to the proposed venotomy site.

11. Either ligate or loosely tie the distal ligature, without cutting the loose ends.

12. While applying traction to the distal tie, nick the vein with a No. 11 scalpel at a 45° angle through ⅓ to ½ of its diameter. Oozing can be controlled by gentle traction on the proximal tie.

13. The mosquito clamp can be used to dilate the vein. The catheter can then be introduced directly into the lumen or through a separate stab wound near the incision site and then into the lumen.

14. Remove all air from the catheter by backflow of blood. Tie the proximal ligature around the vein and intraluminal catheter. The distal ligature can be removed or, if tied, the ends cut. Oozing may occur if the distal ligature is removed instead of tied.

15. Close the skin with a simple running stitch.

16. Affix the catheter to the skin with a stitch and tape all connections.

17. Dress the wound and immobilize the limb as needed.

18. Obtain an x-ray to determine the position of the catheter.

6

DEFIBRILLATION

INTRODUCTION

By the mid-1980s, many experts in the care of cardiac arrest patients had adopted a largely reductionist viewpoint. This viewpoint holds that only a few medical interventions have an effect on survival from cardiac arrest. An impressive body of clinical, epidemiologic, and laboratory data supports this viewpoint. Basic cardiopulmonary resuscitation, for example, unquestionably benefits patients when started early, but when started more than a few minutes after cardiac arrest it acts only to slow the process of dying, and its effectiveness disappears. Several medications, such as calcium chloride, sodium bicarbonate, and isoproterenol, have been observed to be of limited effectiveness or even detrimental, and are no longer mainstays of immediate treatment.

Epidemiologic studies, as well as clinical observations from coronary catheterization laboratories, intensive care units, and cardiac rehabilitation exercise programs, reveal that almost all neurologically intact survivors of out-of-hospital cardiac arrest emerge from a well-defined group of patients: those whose cardiac arrest was witnessed, for whom CPR was started within minutes, who were in ventricular fibrillation, and for whom defibrillation was provided rapidly. The 1986 Standards and Guidelines for Emergency Cardiac Care reflect this reductionist perspective by the repeated observation that the greatest improvement in survival from cardiac arrest will be achieved by a single intervention—early defibrillation.

Because of the primacy of early defibrillation as the most effective intervention for resuscitation of patients from cardiac arrest, a number of new approaches are being tried. These include early defibrillation in the prehospital setting by minimally trained emergency personnel, widespread use of automatic external defibrillators by non–emergency-trained community responders, and even defibrillation by family members and friends of patients at high risk for sudden cardiac death. In addition, the advanced cardiac life support protocols have been altered to reflect the current understanding of the importance of early defibrillation.

This chapter provides an overview of defibrillation, with an emphasis on the early use of defibrillators, proper techniques, ways to enhance defibrillation success, and approaches to refractory

VF. Finally, there is a discussion of future directions in defibrillation.

PHYSIOLOGY OF DEFIBRILLATION

Electrical Principles

The amount of energy (joules or watt-seconds) that reaches the myocardium from a defibrillator is a function of the original potential of the electric charge (volts), the flow of electricity (current or amperes), and the duration of the flow (seconds):

Energy = Potential × Current × Duration
(joules) (volts) (amperes) (seconds)

Another term necessary to understand is electrical power (watts). Power is the product of the voltage and the current:

Power = Potential × Current
(watts) (volts) (amperes)

It is not, however, electrical energy that defibrillates the heart, but *peak electric current*. Unfortunately, defibrillator controls are not set to express the current delivered to the myocardium, but instead display energy, that is, power (watts) delivered over time (joules, or [formerly] watt-seconds). Typically, power in the range of 60,000 watts is discharged over an extremely brief period, such as 4–5 milliseconds, with a resultant energy output of 300 joules (watt-seconds).

The amount of current that flows through the myocardium is dependent upon the resistance (ohms) that exists between the two paddles of the defibrillator:

Current = Potential/Resistance
(amperes) (volts) (ohms)

Defibrillators are described and tested using a standard resistance load of 50 ohms. An energy level of 200 watt-seconds selected on the energy-select switch of a defibrillator means that the defibrillator delivers 200 watt-seconds of energy *only* if the patient's actual transthoracic resistance is equal to 50 ohms. Some recent defibrillators measure the resistance between the two paddles and adjust the capacitor charge so that the actual delivered energy is equal to the setting on the controls.

Decreasing the Resistance

The relationships noted above underscore the importance of lowering the impedance pathway for the defibrillatory shock. A number of factors have been identified that affect the transthoracic impedance to direct current flow:

1. The amount of energy delivered.
2. The area of the paddle electrodes.
3. The conductive interface between the chest wall and the defibrillator paddles.
4. The distance between the defibrillator paddles (in particular, large volumes of air in the lungs between the electrodes).
5. The number of direct current shocks recently delivered.
6. The time interval between shocks (the closer together in time, the lower the impedance).
7. The type of metal used in the electrodes.

There are other, patient-dependent factors that affect resistance, and these will be discussed in a later section. Most of the factors noted above have been extensively studied, and are now reasonably well standardized:

1. Adult Paddle Diameter: 8–9 cm. Larger paddles permit a greater amount of muscle to be depolarized with a lower current density, thus decreasing the possibility of tissue damage. However, if this current density is too low, the defibrillatory discharge will be ineffective.

2. Commercial Electrode Gels (salt-containing coupling agents). In theory, electrode gels should lower the transthoracic impedance to approximately 50 ohm. Evaluations of these products, however, have revealed a great variation in the resultant transthoracic impedance. Occasionally, lubricating gels and ultrasonic gels have been used as defibrillation coupling agents. These are non–salt-containing gels, however, and should not be used for defibrillation. They can increase the transthoracic resistance over 100%. Bare paddles against the skin, however, produce even higher impedance, so if specific defibrillation coupling gel is not available, lubricating or ultrasonic non–salt-containing gels can be substituted.

3. Intrathoracic Volume. Emergency personnel can do little to change the intrathoracic volume of large obese patients, or those with chronic lung disease. However, the phase of ventilation of the subject can be varied by the rescuer. There is a marked increase in the transthoracic impedance to direct defibrillator discharge when subjects are shocked in full inspiration compared with expiration. The transthoracic impedance is decreased by 12% by shock delivery during expiration as compared with inspiration. The obvious recommendation is that the patient's lungs should *not* be inflated during countershock delivery.

4. Paddle Pressure. An additional recommendation is that firm paddle pressure should be applied to the chest to force air from the lungs. This brings the paddles closer together, improves the contact between the skin surface and the paddles, and lowers the transthoracic impedance. The transthoracic impedance is decreased by about 10% by firm paddle pressure. It has been standard to recommend paddle pressures of 25 pounds. Though originally thought to be more effective because of enhanced skin–paddle contact, evidence now suggests that the major benefit of firm paddle pressure is to decrease the amount of air in the lungs between the electrodes.

Recently, adhesive electrodes and conductive adhesives used have been developed for use with the new automatic external defibrillators and transcutaneous pacemakers. Initial evidence suggests that even though there is no firm paddle pressure to squeeze air out of the lungs when these devices are used, they are equally effective at defibrillation when compared with hand-held paddles.

5. Number of Shocks Delivered and Time Period Between Shocks. Transthoracic impedance falls with successive direct current shocks. Recent clinical studies suggest that this decrease in transthoracic impedance is due to skin impregnation by the salt-containing coupling agents, and by an increase in muscle blood flow immediately beneath the paddles. The amount of this decrease is dependent upon the time interval between the shocks. These observations are the rationale behind the current recommendation of the AHA to deliver "stacked" or "serial" shocks. In this approach, when the rhythm is a persistent VF, the defibrillator paddles are not removed from the chest between the second and third countershocks.

"Stacked shocks" are also advocated because of the concept of a critical mass of the myocardium being required to sustain VF. The argument is that the initial countershock may not have defibrillated the entire myocardium; a "critical mass" of myocardium may remain in fibrillation and serve to repropagate VF throughout the entire heart. If the portion of the heart that remains in VF is rapidly shocked a second time, the mass of fibrillating myocardium can be reduced below the critical mass, and VF will not restart. Recent laboratory work, however, suggests that this "critical mass" concept of the fibrillating heart may be incorrect, and that brief isoelectric windows occur even after unsuccessful defibrillatory shocks.

6. Electrode Metal. Various metal alloys such as copper and nickel provide an extremely low transthoracic impedance. Nevertheless, stainless steel is the most commonly used metal on modern defibrillator paddles, because of its lower cost, durability, and inertness.

The Physiologic Basis of Defibrillation

The current delivered by an electric countershock causes the simultaneous depolarization or repolarization—electrophysiologists are not sure which—of much of the ventricular tissue. This renders the myocardium refractory to the conduction of the VF activation wavefronts, and the VF disappears. After this general depolarization of myocardium, an ordered depolarization/repolarization sequence may arise from those pacemaker areas of the heart that possess intrinsic automaticity. Studies have demonstrated that the probability of these natural pacemaker areas of the heart arising after a defibrillatory shock is directly related to how long the heart has been in VF. In addition, the metabolic milieu of the heart muscle, such as its acid/base status, and the degree of oxygenation are critical to the return of natural automaticity.

The current of a defibrillatory shock, in addition to causing a rapid depolarization of the myocardium, will suppress the normal and subsidiary pacemaker areas of the heart both by a direct effect and indirectly by stimulation of a tremendous autonomic discharge. Consequently, if the post-defibrillation rhythm is asystole, there should be an immediate resumption of CPR for one or two cycles. CPR may produce enough coronary artery blood flow to allow the intrinsic pacemaker areas of the heart to recover from the countershock. (See Chapter 8 for a discussion of transcutaneous pacemakers for post-defibrillation asystole.)

DEFIBRILLATORS

The major components and design of defibrillators must be understood to ensure effective defibrillation. Even though defibrillation appears to be a simple procedure, there are many steps in which errors may occur. These errors can either delay shock delivery or completely prevent it.

Waveforms

Though a variety of waveforms have been used in defibrillators, the presently available commercial devices use either a damped half-sinusoidal waveform or a truncated exponential waveform. In theory, the sinusoidal waveform should be less effective at defibrillation of the myocardium. Sinusoidal waveforms have excessively long energy tails, whereas truncated waveform defibrillators arrest the current and voltage waves before a relatively slow decay to zero. The low energy tail of the sinusoidal waveform is thought to occasionally produce refibrillation following the defibrillation of the initial part of the waveform. Though no clinical comparisons of the two types of waveforms have been conducted, animal evaluations have showed no differences between the two devices in defibrillation effectiveness.

Energy

One of the more debated topics in emergency medicine over the past decade has focused on the amount of energy that should be used to defibrillate the heart. There are several points that are now generally accepted:

1. A dose-response curve (that is, a relationship between the subject's weight and the peak current required for defibrillation) does not seem to exist in humans as it does in animals. Rather, the pathway for the defibrillatory energy between the two paddles is the critical factor. The size of the rest of the body does not appear to be significant. The currently recommended dose of 3 joules/kg (200–300 joules) for adults seems adequate.

2. Some histologically detectable myocardial damage occurs with countershocks, but it is minor and relatively unimportant compared with promptly restoring spontaneous circulation.

3. Debate continues over whether post-countershock functional toxicity exists following higher energy levels (>300 joules). The toxic effects of higher energy countershocks include slower recovery of the natural pacemakers, higher degrees of heart block, and more prolonged asystole.

4. Most patients "saved" from VF require only one or two countershocks, delivered at the presently recommended energy level of 200–300 joules. The debate is over what energy level to go to if the rhythm is still VF after two shocks. Stated succinctly: higher energy shocks for resistant VF leave the heart in asystole; lower energy shocks leave the heart in VF.

5. A number of emergency medical systems are now taking the approach of ordering repetitive lower energy shocks (200 joules) for refractory VF, rather than moving to higher energy levels for subsequent shocks. Their rationale is that repetitive shocks will be just as effective at defibrillation of the myocardium, and there will be a higher probability that the post-shock rhythms will be capable of sustaining the circulation. No good data yet exist to confirm whether this approach will result in better survival rates.

Device Controls

All persons who may be called upon to defibrillate a person in cardiac arrest have the responsibility to become familiar with the operating controls of the defibrillator they are likely to use. For emergency personnel in the prehospital setting such knowledge is part of their job responsibility, and equipment and procedure familiarization should be reviewed frequently. The national standard recommended for emergency medical technicians is either clinical use of the defibrillator or a practical skills review every 90 days. The same standard should exist for all physicians, house officers, and nurses who staff emergency rooms, intensive care and coronary care units, or any location where use of a defibrillator is a possibility. Unfortunately, we have frequently observed that failure of house staff and other emergency personnel to be thoroughly acquainted with their equipment is responsible for harmful delays in delivery of defibrillatory shocks.

As a minimum, the following controls should be learned for every defibrillator a rescuer may potentially use:

1. Power-on Switch. Does this switch turn on both the defibrillator and the monitor? Some defibrillators have separate power switches for the monitor/paper recorder and for the actual defibrillator. In addition, check to see whether a *power-on* switch is located on the paddles of the defibrillator. This feature is more often found on portable defibrillators designed for prehospital use.

2. Energy-Select Switch. Check this switch immediately upon turning on the power, and set it at 200 joules if a cardiac arrest is in progress. This is done before assessing the rhythm. When the power is turned off, this switch should be left at the zero position.

3. Charge Button. Most defibrillators have a separate control to initiate charging of the defibrillator capacitors after the energy-select switch has been set. There are some older defibrillators with a meter that permits a continuous range of settings; with these devices, the charge control must be held down until the meter reaches the desired energy setting. Become familiar with how the defibrillator indicates that the capacitors are fully charged and the shock is ready to be delivered. Most frequently, a flashing light or an intermittent tone becomes constant when the full charge is reached. This will take 3–6 seconds on most defibrillators.

4. Discharge Buttons. These are usually located on the defibrillator paddles. Because the paddle handles, however, may also incorporate *power-on* and *energy-select* switches, the operator can become confused and may experience some delay while attempting to locate the discharge buttons. During this delay the charge on the capacitors may have "bled down," and the shock cannot be delivered unless the capacitors are recharged. Often the only clue that this has happened is the flashing charge light that indicates insufficient charge.

5. Lead-Select Switch. This switch is the source of a common error in the management of a cardiac arrest. It must be placed in the "paddle" position when the rhythm is assessed through the "quick-look" feature of some defibrillators; otherwise an accurate rhythm assessment is impossible. The monitor screen will display only what is received through the monitor leads. Since the monitor leads are usually not attached during the initial minutes of a cardiac arrest, only uninterpretable artifact will be displayed. Conversely, rhythms received by the monitor through monitor leads will not be displayed on the screen if the lead-select switch is placed in the "paddles" position.

6. Synchronization Button. In the synchronization mode, the monitor waits to detect an R wave prior to delivery of the electric shock. This R wave must be received through attached monitor leads. Therefore, to perform a synchronized cardioversion, the lead-select switch must be placed in the monitor position, and R waves must be received. In VF, no true R waves are received; consequently, the defibrillator will not deliver shocks to VF in the synchronized mode. VF can be shocked only when the defibrillator is placed in the asynchronous mode. Therefore:

    a. *To shock VF:* The defibrillator *must* be in the *asynchronous mode*; the rhythm signal can be received either through the quick-look paddles or through monitor leads (monitor leads are much more accurate and less prone to artifact).

    b. *To cardiovert:* The defibrillator *must* be in the *synchronized mode*, and the rhythm signal must be received through the monitor leads.

  7. Size of the ECG. Another common error is to have the gain on the monitor display of the ECG rhythm turned up either too low or too high. If the gain is too high, it causes such marked distortion of the signal that it becomes difficult to interpret. If it is too low, it may cause P waves and even QRS complexes to be unrecognized, and a misdiagnosis of asystole may occasionally be made.

THE TECHNIQUE OF DEFIBRILLATION

Defibrillation should not be thought of as simply the proper operation of the defibrillator. The steps of defibrillation are best understood and learned as parts of two cycles.

Step 1: Rhythm Assessment Cycle

The goal of the rhythm assessment cycle is to obtain a proper recording of the patient's cardiac rhythm. Excessive artifact and 60-cycle interference are the most frequent difficulties that interfere with obtaining a clear, interpretable rhythm. Troubleshooting artifact and other problems is discussed in the next section.

  1. Turn the power ON; turn the synchronizer switch OFF; verify that the monitor screen begins to display a signal.

  2. Select the energy level.

  3. Decide on the rhythm assessment method:

    a. *Through the paddles?* Turn the lead selector switch to "paddles" if a quick look at the rhythm through the defibrillator paddles is going to be used, and apply electrode gel to the paddles.

    b. *Through the monitor leads?* If monitor leads are to be used to assess the rhythm (the approach we strongly recommend), turn the lead selector switch to lead I, II, or III. A lead II signal usually provides the best P waves. Attach the adhesive monitor lead patches as follows:

      (1) "White to the right"—the white lead goes to the right shoulder area.

    (2) "Red to the ribs"—the red lead goes to the left lower rib cage.

    (3) "Green (or black) to the left shoulder"—the green or black ground lead goes to the left shoulder area.

4. Cease all contact with the patient and assess the rhythm.

Step 2: The Treatment Cycle

The treatment cycle begins as soon as the operator verifies that a shockable rhythm is present. All activities must be directed toward delivery of electricity to the myocardium as rapidly as possible, proceeding as follows:

1. Apply electrode gel to the paddles, if not already done.

2. Charge the defibrillator to the selected energy level, using the paddle charge controls.

3. Apply the defibrillator paddles to the chest in the proper position; apply firm pressure against the chest to reduce lung volume and electric resistance.

4. Check that no personnel are touching the patient, and announce that a shock is about to be delivered. The following statements may be helpful: "I'm going to shock on three. Everybody clear the patient. One, two, three."

5. Press both shock delivery buttons simultaneously.

6. Observe for a visible response of the patient to the shock.

7. DO NOT REMOVE THE DEFIBRILLATOR PADDLES FROM THE CHEST: IMMEDIATELY PRESS THE CHARGE BUTTONS TO RECHARGE THE CAPACITORS. (There will be a 3–5 second period before the monitor screen properly displays the rhythm after a countershock. The defibrillator should be recharged during this time.)

8. REASSESS THE RHYTHM FOR THE CONTINUED PRESENCE OF VF. Check for a pulse if a non-VF rhythm appears. Deliver the second countershock as outlined above.

9. Deliver the second countershock as outlined above.

10. Deliver the third countershock in the same manner if the rhythm is still a shockable one. *REMEMBER: The defibrillator paddles never leave the chest while up to three countershocks are delivered.*

11. After a change in the rhythm, or after the third countershock, proceed with the treatment protocols as outlined in Chapter 10.

TROUBLESHOOTING

Emergency personnel must learn to recognize the most common problems that can occur while attempting to treat patients in

Table 6–1. MOST COMMON
ERRORS IN DEFIBRILLATION

1. Other patient care activities are performed before defibrillation.
2. An accurate and interpretable rhythm is not obtained.
3. Paddle movement artifact is misinterpreted as VF when quick-look paddles are used to assess the rhythm.
4. Lead selector switch is placed in the wrong setting for the chosen method of rhythm assessment.
5. Paddles are placed incorrectly on the chest.
6. The first two or three shocks are not "stacked."
7. Conductive gel is not readily available.
8. The defibrillator charge is allowed to bleed down by delays between charging the defibrillator and delivery of the shock.

cardiac arrest with a defibrillator. Each of these problems should trigger a mental checklist of possible causes and possible solutions. Some of the most common errors observed in defibrillation are outlined in Table 6–1. In this chapter we place a great deal of emphasis upon obtaining a clear rhythm recording through adhesive monitor leads. Rescue personnel in both the hospital and the prehospital setting should not rely upon quick-look defibrillator paddles to accurately assess the rhythm. The advantages of an accurate rhythm tracing far outweigh the disadvantages of the few seconds it takes to attach adhesive monitor electrodes. This means, however, that monitor leads must be readily available and properly used.

Excessive Artifact

Unsnapped Monitor Leads. There are several causes of excessive artifact, but probably the most common is unsnapped monitor leads. This can produce either an artifactually straight line or a monitor screen full of irregular signals. Quickly check to see that the leads are snapped to the adhesive patches whenever excessive artifact is observed. (Unsnapped leads have a tendency to produce an artifactual rhythm that looks distressingly like VF. Virtually everyone in emergency medicine has had the experience of rushing into a patient's room after observing VF on the monitor screen, only to find the smiling face of a completely alert and conscious patient.)

Poor Monitor Lead–Skin Contact. Poor contact between the adhesive monitor patches and the patient's skin is yet another problem that leads to excessive artifact. The first response should always be to push firmly against the monitor patches to see if proper contact can be established. Common causes of this problem include:

1. *Hairy chests.* A small safety razor can be used to quickly shave a small area of the chest.

2. *Sweaty, wet, or dirty chests.* Cardiac patients are often extremely diaphoretic. They may also be wet from rain or from

immersion. Dirt or oil from occupational or other activities may be present. Alcohol swabs for cleaning oil and dirt, 4 × 4 inch gauze, or a small towel to dry off the chest should be available.

3. *Small, bony, or irregular chests.* The monitor leads should be quickly repositioned on the arms or clavicles, or on another portion of the chest.

4. *Dry or defective monitor patches.* The monitor patches can become outdated. Over time, the electrode gel on the patches can evaporate. Expired patches should be replaced. For the acute emergency need, a small amount of the electrode gel can be applied under the patches.

Monitor Cable Movement. The most common causes of monitor cable movement are:

1. Patient movement during transport, either in rescue vehicles, or in the hospital. NEVER attempt to assess the rhythm during any form of patient transport.

2. Agonal respirations or muscle tremor. Often the agonal respirations are spaced far enough apart to permit proper rhythm assessment. Otherwise, the rescue personnel must continue CPR and other features of the resuscitation until the agonal respirations cease.

3. Continued chest compressions or ventilations. All contact with the patient must cease while the rhythm is being assessed.

Excessive 60-Cycle Interference. This is more commonly a problem for prehospital emergency personnel. It can also occur, however, in emergency rooms and coronary care units when improperly shielded or grounded equipment is in use. In the prehospital setting, 60-cycle interference is most often due to nearby electrical appliances, such as electric blankets, fluorescent lights, clocks, and televisions and radios. These appliances should be unplugged, or the patient should be moved to a different location.

SPECIAL TOPICS AND FUTURE DIRECTION

The Precordial Thump and Cough Cardioversion

The precordial thump is a dramatic maneuver that possesses a peculiar popularity with lay rescuers. The maneuver was once taught as part of basic CPR and first aid classes. However, concern over the possibility of conversion of a relatively benign rhythm into a more malignant one led to an abandonment of the precordial thump as a basic CPR maneuver. The 1986 AHA Standards continue the recommendation of the 1980 Standards: Use precordial thump only at the onset of VF or VTACH for patients with a witnessed cardiac arrest, and for whom a backup defibrillator is available.

This recommendation seems eminently reasonable for emergency personnel in hospital settings. There remains, however, a dilemma for prehospital rescue personnel who arrive on the scene of a patient who has recently collapsed from apparent cardiac arrest. Should a precordial thump be given as the very first therapeutic maneuver upon arrival at the scene? How often will the thump convert a patient in ventricular tachycardia to VF? Few studies have data that address these questions. Evidence from Brighton, England, however, suggests that fears that worse rhythms may be induced with the precordial thump are inappropriate. Chamberlain and his colleagues have recommended the following:

1. All conscious patients with VTACH should be asked to cough forcibly.

2. Those who do not respond should be given a precordial thump only if the arrhythmia demands urgent action; adequate explanation should be given, and a backup defibrillator should always be available.

3. All unmonitored patients who develop a verified and witnessed cardiac arrest should receive a "blind" precordial thump.

Countershock of Asystole and Fine VF

A misunderstanding has crept into some emergency medical publications—the concept of "jump-starting" the asystolic heart with an electric shock. A moment of reflection will reveal how irrational such a concept is. The entire purpose of the countershock is to *produce asystole* or complete electrical depolarization. This is done with the expectation that some intrinsic pacemaker tissue in the heart will resume more normal conduction and contraction. If the myocardium is already asystolic, there is clearly no purpose served by delivery of a countershock. This additional electric energy can serve only to further depress intrinsic cardiac automaticity.

There does exist, however, the entity of "occult VF," or VF that "masquerades" as asystole. This condition was first noted in animal studies, but there have also been rare case reports of humans who have had multi-lead ECG tracings obtained during a cardiac arrest, and while some of the leads record asystole, several others record VF. These observations in animals and rarely in humans have led to speculation that an electrical vector exists for VF, especially VF of short duration. VF may not always be caused by numerous small re-entrant pathways, but may occur with large irregular waves of depolarization. The orientation of these waves of depolarization, or vectors of VF, may vary with the site of the initiating stimulus. The result is that VF may masquerade as asystole if only one lead is monitored.

The frequency with which this phenomenon occurs, however, is extremely low. Observations from EMT defibrillation programs in King County, Washington, and in Iowa suggest that occult VF is present in fewer than 1 out of every 200 patients who upon arrival of emergency personnel display asystole. "Asystole" is much more likely to be caused by equipment problems or ineffective patient monitor connections than by occult VF that masquerades as asystole. In addition, because of dismal survival rates, the rhythm "fine VF" (VF with an average amplitude of 3 mm or less on the ECG strip) may more appropriately be classified as asystole.

If an extremely low amplitude or flat line ECG is recorded during a cardiac arrest, the following "asystole protocol" should be followed:

1. Check all monitor cable connections to the patient: Press the monitor patches firmly against the chest, check for conductive gel, check the cable snaps.

2. Check all monitor cable connections at the defibrillator.

3. Check the ECG calibrations of the device, or the ECG size control.

4. Check the power supply.

5. Switch the monitoring electrodes 90 degrees from the original position; this may be done in any one of the following ways:

    a. The lead selector switch can be used to record 5–10 seconds of the rhythm in leads II, III, and I.

    b. The monitor cables can be switched where they are attached to the patient's chest.

    c. The monitoring defibrillator paddles can be placed in different locations on the patient's chest.

If VF is observed with any of these maneuvers, proceed with the standard defibrillation protocols.

Automatic External Defibrillators

Automatic external defibrillators represent the addition of the technique for analysis and interpretation of surface electrocardiographic signals to portable, direct-current defibrillators. The earliest automatic external defibrillators contained analog circuitry, and responded primarily to the rate of the electrical signal. Presently available devices incorporate sophisticated digital software, with algorithms that analyze multiple features of the surface electrocardiographic signal. There are two general approaches to automatic rhythm analysis: time domain techniques and frequency domain techniques. Time domain techniques analyze some combination of the amplitude, frequency, and morphology of a filtered electrocardiographic signal. In the frequency domain approach, a transformation of the electrical signal is performed, and the frequency content and power spectrum of the signal is then analyzed.

Signal verification approaches include measurement of the impedance between the two surface electrodes to verify that there is adequate contact and the absence of motion; filters and masks to identify electrical artifact; and QRS analyzers to verify the absence of sinus or other supraventricular rhythms. The devices record the surface electrocardiographic signal through two adhesive electrode pads, usually placed in a lead II configuration of right sternum and cardiac apex. Defibrillatory shocks are also delivered through these electrodes. Surface electrocardiographic signals are not optimal for analysis by an automatic detector, because they are prone to signal and movement artifact. Nevertheless, at the present time surface signals remain the most practical approach to rapid rhythm analysis.

When an automatic external defibrillator is used in a cardiac arrest, the rescuer must cease contact with the patient while the device assesses the rhythm, charges the capacitor, and delivers countershocks of 200–360 joules of delivered energy. Depending on the manufacturer, the time required for rhythm analysis can range from 6 to 20 seconds, and capacitor charge time from 4 to 11 seconds. There are two general types of automatic external defibrillators: "fully automatic" and "shock-advisory" or "semi-automatic." The fully automatic devices, once attached and turned on, assess the rhythm, charge the capacitors, and deliver countershocks as long as the rhythm remains ventricular fibrillation (VF) or rapid pulseless ventricular tachycardia, or until the device is switched off. The shock-advisory devices require responses by the operator, guided by messages displayed on a liquid crystal screen. If the rhythm is ventricular fibrillation or rapid pulseless ventricular tachycardia, a final step is required in which the operator is "advised" to press the shock button.

Automatic external defibrillators are an exciting development in cardiology. Their simplicity of use, ease of training, and easy portability make them the ideal device for many prehospital personnel such as emergency medical technicians in rural areas. In addition, these devices will be used more frequently by minimally trained community responders located in senior centers, exercise rehabilitation facilities, high-rise office buildings, commercial airplane flights of long duration, and densely populated or remote industrial sites such as work camps, oil rigs, and ships at sea.

Automatic Defibrillators and Emergency Personnel

Emergency personnel should be aware that an increasing percentage of the people they will treat for emergency cardiac problems will have either an automatic implantable defibrillator (AID) placed within their body or a personal automatic external defibrillator (AED) and family members and friends who are trained to use the device in the event of a cardiac arrest. Both types of automatic defibrillators are undergoing intensive clinical evaluations. The evidence so far is that the devices work, that family members can be trained to use the AED, that even though

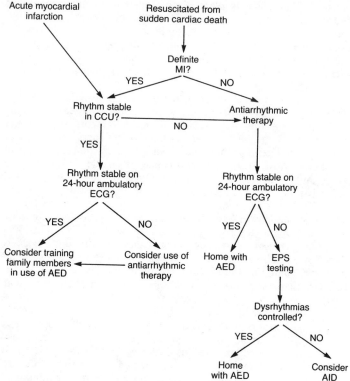

Figure 6–1. Approach to determine candidates for automatic external defibrillators (AEDs) or automatic implantable defibrillators (AIDs).

retention of skills is a slight problem, family members will use the devices at the time of a cardiac arrest, and that they can save lives.

Determination of Candidates for an AED or an AID

All patients who have been resuscitated from sudden cardiac death should be considered for either home placement of an AED or implantation of an AID. In addition, a strong argument can be made that all survivors of a myocardial infarction are candidates for an AED because of their increased risk for lethal dysrhythmias, especially in the first year after their heart attack. Figure 6–1 presents a possible approach to determine which patients should be considered for AEDs and which for AIDs.

REFERENCES

1. American Heart Association: The 1985 standards and guidelines for cardiopulmonary resuscitation (CPR) and emergency cardiac care (ECC). JAMA 255:2905, 1986.
2. Caldwell G, Millar G, Quinn E, et al: Simple mechanical methods for cardioversion: defence of the precordial thump and cough version. Br. Med J 291:627, 1985.
3. Weaver WD, Cobb LA, Dennis D, et al: Amplitude of ventricular fibrillation waveform and outcome after cardiac arrest. Ann Intern Med 102:53, 1985.
4. Weaver WD, Cobb LA, Copass MK, et al: Ventricular defibrillation—a comparative trial using 185-J and 320-J shocks. N Engl J Med 307:1101, 1982.
5. Ewy GA, Dahl CF, Zimmerman M, et al: Ventricular fibrillation masquerading as ventricular standstill. Crit Care Med 12:841, 1981.
6. McDonald JL: Coarse ventricular fibrillation presenting as asystole or very low amplitude ventricular fibrillation. Crit Care Med 10:790, 1982.
7. Gauscho JA, Crampton RS, Cherwek ML, et al.: Determinants of ventricular defibrillation in adults. Circulation 60:231, 1979.
8. Ornato JP, Gonzalez ER: Refractory ventricular fibrillation. Emerg Decisions 2:35, 1986.
9. Vassale M: On the mechanisms underlying cardiac standstill: factors determining success or failure of escape pacemakers in the heart. J Am Coll Cardiol 5:35B, 1985.
10. Cummins RO, Eisenberg MS, Hearne TR, et al: Automatic external defibrillation: evaluations of its role in the home and in emergency medical systems. Ann Emerg Med 13(Part 2):798, 1984.
11. Surawicz B: Ventricular fibrillation. J Am Coll Cardiol 1985;5:43B, 1985.
12. Ewy GA: Defibrillation. In Harwood AL (ed): Cardiopulmonary Resuscitation. Baltimore, Williams & Wilkins, 1982, pp 89–126.
13. Greenberg MI, Hedges JR: Defibrillation. In Roberts JR, Hedges JR (eds): Clinical procedures in emergency medicine. Philadelphia, WB Saunders, 1985, pp 160–169.
14. Safar P: Cardiopulmonary cerebral resuscitation: basic and advanced life support. In Schwartz GR, Safar P, Stone JH, et al (eds): Principles and Practice of Emergency Medicine, 2nd ed. Philadelphia, WB Saunders, 1985, pp. 277–282.
15. Cummins RO, Eisenberg MS: Automatic external defibrillators: clinical issues for cardiology. Circulation 73:381, 1986.
16. Stults KR, Brown DD: Converting asystole. J Emerg Med Serv 9:38, 1984.
17. Eisenberg MS, Hallstrom AP, Copass MK, et al: Treatment of out-of-hospital cardiac arrest with rapid defibrillation by emergency medical technicians. N Engl J Med 302:1379, 1980.
18. Stults KR, Brown DD, Kerber RE: Efficacy of an automated external defibrillator in the management of out-of-hospital cardiac arrest: validation of the diagnostic algorithm and initial clinical experience in a rural environment. Circulation 1986;73:701, 1986.
19. Weaver WD, Copass MK, Hill DL, et al: Cardiac arrest treated with a new automatic external defibrillator by out-of-hospital first responders. Am J Cardiol 57:1017, 1986.
20. Cummins RO, Eisenberg MS, Litwin PE, et al: Automatic external defibrillators used by emergency medical technicians. JAMA 257:1605, 1987.

7

ADDITIONAL TECHNIQUES

The procedures described below should be performed by nonspecialists only in the event of a cardiac arrest or imminent cardiac arrest when specialists are not immediately available. Thus, only emergency techniques are described. The same procedures when performed electively may require different techniques, equipment, or supplies.

PERICARDIOCENTESIS

Pericardiocentesis is a dangerous procedure with high risks of catastrophic complications, such as laceration of the coronary artery, laceration of the myocardium, and induction of fatal arrhythmias. However, it can be both diagnostic and lifesaving when performed during a cardiac arrest in a patient with possible cardiac tamponade. It should be performed in all unsuccessful resuscitations where electrical mechanical dissociation (EMD) is present and hypovolemia and tension pneumothorax are either absent or have already been treated.

Equipment and Supplies:
1. Material for skin sterilization and sterile gloves if time permits
2. Syringe, 30–50 ml
3. Pericardiocentesis needle, usually an 18-gauge spinal needle
4. Conductive cable with alligator clamps on each end (optional)
5. Specimen tubes, lavender-topped (with anticoagulant) and red-topped

Procedure:
1. The operator should stand facing the supine patient on the patient's right side.
2. If available and a QRS complex is present, attach one alligator clamp of the cable to the chest lead of the electrocardiograph and the other clamp to the metal hub of the needle (if the hub is plastic, attach the clamp to the needle, near the hub). Turn the setting of the electrocardiograph to the V-lead. An injury pattern (ST elevation) will be seen if the needle contacts the myocardium.
3. Sterilize the skin around the patient's xiphoid, avoiding interruption of CPR if possible. Observe as much sterile technique as time permits (e.g., gloves).
4. Stop CPR and proceed rapidly with the steps below.
5. Insert the needle through the skin at a 30–45° angle to the

skin just to the left of the xiphoid (see Fig. 7–1). Remove the stylet and attach the syringe. Piercing the skin without the stylet may cause occlusion of the lumen of the needle by a skin plug and give a false negative pericardiocentesis result.

6. While pulling back continuously on the plunger of the syringe, advance the needle toward the patient's sternal notch.

7. If fluid or blood is aspirated into the syringe, withdraw as much as possible or as allowed by the size of the syringe. In acute tamponade, withdrawal of as little as 10 ml of pericardial fluid can cause a dramatic hemodynamic improvement. The source of the blood (pericardial vs. intracardiac) can often be determined by the fact that pericardial blood does not clot.

8. If no fluid is aspirated, withdraw the needle to just under the skin and redirect the needle medially.

9. Be sure not to interrupt chest compression by greater than 30–45 seconds if pericardiocentesis is not the final procedure.

10. Pericardial aspiration can also be performed via an approach at the 4th intercostal space along the left sternal border, with the needle advancing perpendicular to the chest. This approach should be tried only as a last resort, because of the greater risk of complications.

11. After aspiration is completed, withdraw the needle and apply direct pressure over the site.

12. Resume CPR as indicated.

13. If the patient's hemodynamic status improves, definitive therapy can be performed by specialists in the operating room or fluoroscopy suite.

INTRACARDIAC INJECTION

Intracardiac administration of drugs is not recommended if a central intravenous line can be inserted. The high risk of complications associated with intracardiac injection (cardiac tamponade, laceration of myocardium, laceration of coronary artery, induction of fatal arrhythmia) negates any possible advantage over administration of drugs via a central line. However, if a central line cannot be established within a reasonable time, and resuscitation is unsuccessful, intracardiac administration of drugs can be used as a last resort.

Equipment and Supplies:
1. Material for skin sterilization
2. Prepackaged, prefilled syringe with intracardiac injection needle, or syringe with drug to be administered attached to a spinal needle

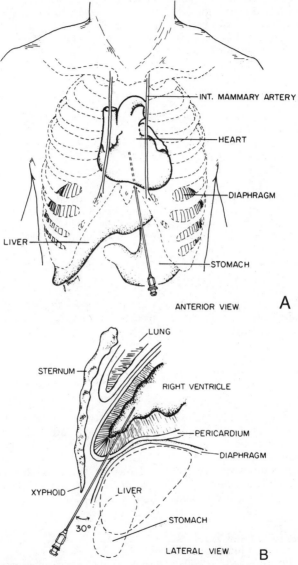

Figure 7–1. Subxyphoid approach to the right ventricle. *A*, Frontal view. *B*, Lateral view. Note proximity of stomach and liver to entrance point. (From Roberts JR, Hedges JR: Clinical Procedures in Emergency Medicine. Philadelphia, WB Saunders, 1985, p. 197. Reprinted with permission.)

Procedure:
1. Sterilize the skin over the patient's xiphoid.
2. Flush out all air from the syringe and needle.
3. Stop chest compressions.
4. Insert the needle to the left of the xiphoid at a 30–45° angle to the skin. While pulling back on the plunger, advance the needle toward the patient's sternal notch.
5. When blood is aspirated into the syringe, inject the contents of the syringe and immediately withdraw the needle.
6. Resume chest compressions.

8

EMERGENCY CARDIAC PACING: TRANSCUTANEOUS PACING, TRANSVENOUS PACING, AND TRANSTHORACIC PACING

Several studies have compared the transcutaneous pacemaker approach with either the transvenous or the transthoracic approach in the emergency setting. Table 8–1 compares several features of the three approaches to emergency pacing. These studies have established the transcutaneous approach to be equally successful in achieving both electrical and mechanical "capture" of the cardiac rhythm. The equivalent effectiveness, noninvasiveness, and marked superiority in speed and ease of use of the transcutaneous pacemaker clearly make it the pacing technique of choice for the emergency treatment of asystole and profound bradycardias.

Because of the relative newness of the approach, this chapter concentrates upon transcutaneous pacing. Successful transcutaneous pacing, however, must be followed by more definitive care. This means that the next step for a patient who experiences a perfusing, pacemaker-dependent rhythm will be transvenous or transthoracic pacing. The techniques of transvenous and transthoracic pacing are discussed at the end of the chapter for those emergency situations in which transcutaneous pacing is unavailable, unsuccessful, or must be followed by another approach.

TRANSCUTANEOUS PACEMAKERS

Transcutaneous cardiac pacing (alternatively referred to as "non-invasive pacing") is a rapidly applied and noninvasive technique for the treatment of asystole and severe bradycardias. Early transcutaneous pacemakers from the 1950s produced several problems that prevented clinical acceptance. These included painful external stimulation of the skin and muscles, and superficial ulcerations under the chest electrodes. The transcutaneous approach to pacing was temporarily abandoned in the 1960s with the development of the implantable pacemaker and improvements in transvenous techniques. However, the following recent advances in technology and design allowed engineers to overcome the problems associated with the first-generation transcutaneous pacemakers:

1. Larger surface electrodes plus a high-impedance conductive medium between the electrodes and the skin were developed. The

higher-impedance conductive material spreads the energy out more, making it less concentrated and thus causing less pain. This permits the pacing stimulus amplitude to be lowered and helps to reduce the sharp pain that results from electrical stimulation of surface nerves.

2. The duration of the pacing stimulus was lengthened. This decreases the amount of current required for electrical capture and consequently the amount of skeletal muscle contraction. The pain of transcutaneous pacing in a conscious patient is caused by two features: (1) the electricity going into the skin, which can be reduced as noted above, and (2) the skeletal muscle contractions from the electrical stimulus. Little can be done to reduce the pain due to skeletal muscle contraction.

The recent development of commercially available transcutaneous pacemakers has stimulated much clinical research in this technique. At the present time these devices have achieved little success with patients in asystole, primarily because of long delays between the cardiac arrest and application of the device, and failure to try transcutaneous pacing until all other resuscitative methods have failed. Transcutaneous pacemakers have, however, been demonstrated to be useful clinically in patients with pulsatile bradycardias, and occasionally in patients with idioventricular rhythms.

Equipment

Demand, Synchronous, and Asynchronous Pacemakers

Implanted cardiac pacemakers have become the standard and are an effective approach to many rhythm disorders. Certain terms are used in reference to implanted pacemakers that do not always apply to transcutaneous pacemakers:

1. *Demand pacemakers* deliver a stimulus whenever the heart rate falls below a certain preset rate. The pacing stimulus can be "asynchronous" if it occurs at any point in the cardiac cycle, such as on the R wave or the T wave. The currently available transcutaneous pacemakers have a demand mode.

2. *Synchronous pacemakers* synchronize the stimulus with some feature of the patient's natural rhythm, such as the P or the R wave. Not all of the currently available transcutaneous pacemakers have a synchronous mode.

3. *Asynchronous pacemakers* are set to deliver a stimulus at a set rate. They do not "synch" with any feature of the electrocardiographic signal, and do not respond to the patient's intrinsic rate.

In general, when transcutaneous pacemakers are used to pace patients with a bradycardia, they are set in a *synchronized demand* mode. When they are used to pace patients with asystole they are set in the *asynchronous mode*.

Table 8–1. COMPARATIVE FEATURES OF TRANSVENOUS, TRANSTHORACIC, AND TRANSCUTANEOUS PACEMAKERS

Feature	Transvenous	Transthoracic	Transcutaneous
Location of Use:	Hospital only	Hospital only	Pre-hospital or in hospital
Procedural Time Prior to Pacing:	10–15 minutes	3–5 minutes	½ to 2 minutes
Type of Procedure:	Invasive through central veins	Invasive through chest wall	Noninvasive
Skill Level:	Highly skilled procedure	Highly skilled procedure	Simple
Complication Rates:	14–20%	10–20%	Few and minor
Potential Complications:	Arterial puncture Pneumothorax Thrombophlebitis Infection/sepsis R ventricle perforation Pulmonary embolism Cardiac tamponade Failure after countershocks	Lung puncture Pneumothorax Internal bleeding Infection/sepsis Coronary artery laceration Cardiac tamponade Dysrhythmias Failure with electrode displacement	Skin erythema
Disadvantages:	High complication rates 35–40% malfunction rate Not portable	High complication rates Emergencies only Not portable	Some discomfort Pulse difficult to palpate owing to muscle contractions
Contraindications:	Patients on anticoagulants or streptokinase	Patients on anticoagulants or streptokinase	Open chest wounds

(Based upon a table from Wiegel A, White RD: Non-invasive pacing: a pre-hospital ALS alternative. J Emerg Med Services *10*:35, 1985. Used with permission.)

Pacing Electrodes

In transcutaneous cardiac pacing, two pregelled adhesive electrodes are applied to the patient's chest, either one anteriorly and one posteriorly, or one at the lower left anterior ribs and the other at the upper right sternal border. Pacing is initiated by delivery of current through the electrodes, which are attached to a portable pulse generator. There are currently four commercially available transcutaneous pacemakers. Two of these pacemakers combine transcutaneous pacing with a defibrillator. One device incorporates a pacemaker with an automatic external monitor/defibrillator, and can deliver pacing stimuli through the same adhesive electrodes used to deliver defibrillatory shocks.

The conducting surface of the electrodes in some devices is bordered by an adhesive rim. In other products the electrode itself is a "conductive adhesive" in which the entire surface adheres to the skin and conducts electricity.

Device Controls

Four pacing parameters determine the effectiveness of transcutaneous pacing:

1. The current delivered (milliamperes)
2. The duration of the current (milliseconds)
3. The rate of current delivery (pulses per minute)
4. The surface area of the skin over which the current is delivered (usually at least 8 cm diameter)

The presently available devices deliver operator-adjusted currents from 0 to 200 milliamperes (measured against a 50-ohm test load), at pulse durations of 20–40 milliseconds (not operator-adjustable), and at variable or fixed rates of up to 180 beats per minute.

Rhythm Display

Monitor leads from the electrocardiogram are placed on the chest wall and attached to a special electrocardiogram that is either built into the pacemaker pulse generator or separately attached. Standard electrocardiogram monitors or recorders are overloaded by the strong pacing stimulus of the device, and their display of the paced rhythm is usually uninterpretable. The electrocardiographic devices built to accompany transcutaneous pacers incorporate special circuitry within their detection systems that enables monitoring of the heart's response to the pacing stimulus.

Electrical and Mechanical Capture

Two terms must be defined and understood in any discussion of transcutaneous pacing. Unfortunately, authors frequently ignore this requirement, and the results presented in several articles about transcutaneous pacing are uninterpretable.

1. Electrical Capture. Electrical capture means that the stimulus from the pacemaker either stimulates some natural pacemaker in the heart, such as the SA or AV node, or directly stimulates the normal conducting pathways in the myocardium. This impulse must produce both depolarization and subsequent repolarization. Successful electrical capture should be defined as: (a) a resultant QRS complex of at least 0.14 msec (not to be confused with the narrow, sometimes QRS-like artifact of the pacing stimulus itself); (b) a T wave that follows the paced complex; and (c) disappearance of the underlying rhythm.

2. Mechanical Capture. Mechanical capture means that the muscle of the heart has been stimulated to contract, and this myocardial contraction must produce a palpable pulse. The stimulation for this contraction may have occurred through the normal conducting tissues of the heart; hence, the above criteria for electrical capture will be met. This would be termed a combination of electrical and mechanical capture. The contraction may also have occurred because of direct electrical stimulus to the myocardium, and therefore the signal complex will be broad. This would be termed mechanical capture without electrical capture. Palpation at the carotid artery is the most sensitive location to detect a palpable pulse and determine if mechanical capture has occurred. However, the skeletal muscle contractions that occur with transcutaneous pacing can easily confuse the person who attempts carotid palpation. In several studies true mechanical capture has been difficult to establish, because a reportedly palpable pulse has not always been accompanied by a measurable blood pressure.

Indications for Transcutaneous Pacemakers

The indications for transcutaneous pacing are discussed below and are summarized in Table 8–2.

1. Symptomatic Bradycardias (unresponsive to atropine). These are defined as heart rates of 40 or below that result in signs of decreased cardiac output, such as altered level of consciousness, hypotension, congestive heart failure, shortness of breath, or chest pain. Symptomatic bradycardias can occur in a large variety of clinical situations, both with and without acute myocardial infarction.

2. Asymptomatic Bradycardias (prophylactic placement of pacing pads). Two of the most frequent uses of transcutaneous pacemakers are (1) for patients who are bradycardic from high-degree heart block or digitalis toxicity but are not yet symptomatic and thus do not need external pacing, and (2) for patients who are awaiting placement of a permanent or temporary transvenous pacemaker. The pacing pads can be attached to the patient and the device readied for immediate operation, but not actually turned

Table 8–2. INDICATIONS FOR TRANSCUTANEOUS PACEMAKERS

1. **Symptomatic Bradycardias** (unresponsive to atropine with HR <40)
   - AV block
   - Sinus node dysfunction
   - Drug toxicity (verapamil, digoxin)
   - Pacemaker function, implanted
   - Hyperkalemia
2. **Asymptomatic Bradycardias** (prophylactic placement of pacing pads)
   - Same clinical situations noted above
   - During cardiac catheterizations
   - Induction of anesthesia
3. **Asystole (Ventricular Standstill)**
4. **Pulseless Idioventricular Rhythm (PIVR)**
5. **Post-Defibrillation Asystole**
6. **Overdrive Pacing**
   - Recurrent VF
   - Atrial tachycardias
   - Ventricular tachycardias
   - Torsades de pointes

on unless symptoms develop. Many transient heart blocks and drug toxicities may resolve with the device never having to be used.

3. Asystole (Ventricular Standstill). Noninvasive pacing must be used within minutes of the onset of asystole. The device should be attached and readied the moment asystole is identified, rather than awaiting other interventions such as intubation and initiation of central venous lines (see Table 8–2). There are few reports of electrical and mechanical capture for patients in asystole more than 10 minutes.

4. Pulseless Idioventricular Rhythm (PIVR). The prospect for success is somewhat greater for this ill-defined rhythm than for asystole; however, the same caveats about *early use* apply. External pacing must be attempted within minutes of the onset of PIVR for there to be any possibility of success.

5. Post-Defibrillation Asystole. Asystole that follows an electrical countershock is, in effect, only seconds old. In theory, the best prospect for successful transcutaneous pacing lies with this very large subset of cardiac arrest patients. In prehospital care, close to 50% of the patients initially in VF are shocked into asystole. Immediate transcutaneous pacing in this situation may have some positive benefit, although controlled, prospective studies have not yet confirmed this possibility.

6. Overdrive Pacing. As discussed in Chapter 6, Defibrillation, there are occasional patients in VF who can be defibrillated but who then return to VF. Most often this problem of refibrillation can be solved by further countershocks, by antifibrillatory medications, or by intubation. Emergency personnel should be aware that if the rhythm between episodes of VF is a brady-dysrhythmia (such as asystole, idioventricular rhythm, or bradycardia), over-drive pacing by a transcutaneous pacemaker may be effective in prevention of refibrillation. In addition, there have been reports of successful use of overdrive transcutaneous pacing for atrial tachycardias, ventricular tachycardias, and torsades de pointes.

Recommended Procedure for Bradyasystolic Cardiac Arrest

The Importance of Early Use of Transcutaneous Pacing

Table 8–3 and Figure 8–1 present our recommended procedure for the use of transcutaneous pacing in cardiac arrest patients. Emergency personnel will note that this procedure differs in sequencing from the AHA recommended guidelines. The AHA recommends that early pacing "be considered" after endotracheal intubation, after intravenous lines have been established, and after epinephrine and atropine have been administered.

Our recommendation is to initiate transcutaneous pacing as soon as the initial assessment of the rhythm reveals asystole, profound bradycardia, or pulseless idioventricular rhythm. This does not mean that intubation or administration of medications should be delayed while pacing is attempted. Instead the rescuers should, as much as is practical, proceed *simultaneously* with these interventions. The dynamics of an actual arrest permit multiple rescuers to work in concert: while one rescuer prepares the intravenous line, another prepares to intubate, and a third attaches the transcutaneous monitor/pacing electrodes.

Single-Rescuer Sequence for Transcutaneous Pacing

If there is only one rescuer with advanced life support skills present at the resuscitation attempt, our recommendation is the following sequence of interventions (this assumes CPR has been initiated and is continued at all possible times):

1. Assess the rhythm:
   a. If VF: defibrillate.
   b. If asystole, PIVR, or bradycardia <40 BPM: initiate transcutaneous pacing.
2. Perform endotracheal intubation; administer epinephrine endotracheally (pacing continues while intubation is performed).
3. Establish intravenous line and administer indicated medications.

Complications

Transcutaneous pacemakers can produce little additional harm to patients in complete cardiac arrest from asystole or PIVR. Complications will occur in patients who have significant bradycar-

Table 8–3. RECOMMENDED PROCEDURE FOR USE OF
TRANSCUTANEOUS PACEMAKERS IN BRADYASYSTOLIC ARREST
(see Figure 8–1)

1. Confirm cardiopulmonary arrest.
2. Initiate or continue CPR.
3. Assess the rhythm by monitor leads or "quick-look" paddles.
4. Connect external pacemaker immediately if the rhythm is:
   a. Asystole
   b. Pulseless idioventricular rhythm (PIVR) (<40 bpm).
   c. Sinus or junctional bradycardias (<40 bpm).
5. Place the anterior and posterior pacing electrodes on the patient. (Attach monitor electrodes to the patient if recommended by the manufacturer.)
6. Set rate at 80 ppm, turn power on, turn pacing on, and start with current output at 70–80 milliamperes. If capture of the rhythm does not occur, gradually increase output up to the highest current setting on the device, as needed. (*Note*: There are several clinical states that may elevate the pacing threshold of the mycoardium: hypoxia, cardiomyopathy, emphysema, heavy thoracic musculature, obesity, and a long period of arrest prior to pacing, especially if there has been no CPR during this period.)
7. Carotid or femoral pulses should be checked to determine response to pacing. Successful mechanical capture is almost always detectable by a *femoral pulse*. Palpation of the carotid pulse *without* a femoral pulse during pacing usually indicates failed mechanical capture with palpation of muscle contraction artifact at the neck. Palpation of pulses should at some point be confirmed by a measured blood pressure; however, the resuscitation should not be delayed for cuff placement, etc.
8. Observe the monitor for pacemaker output. Identification of successful pacing may be difficult, owing to the large pacer spike and artifact from patient movement. If a pulse returns with pacing, reduce current output to just above threshold. Continue to check for a pulse. Leave the sensitivity of the device in the asynchronous position.
9. If electrical capture occurs, but without a palpable pulse, CPR with chest compressions should be continued simultaneously with pacing for at least 1 minute and then the pulse rechecked.
10. If a pulse is generated by pacing, immediately start an IV line and insert an endotracheal tube. Check BP; if less than 60 mm Hg, resume CPR.
11. When a palpable pulse is generated during pacing, interrupt pacing every 2–3 minutes for 10 seconds, and check for a spontaneous pulse. If there is no pulse, resume pacing and simultaneous chest compressions.
12. If there is no response to maximum pacing output (150–200 milliamperes and rate up to 120 bpm), stop pacing and proceed with the standard protocol, including IV line, endotracheal intubation, and CPR.
13. Pacing electrodes should remain in place while awaiting any response to drug therapy. Intermittently check for capture by turning the pacemaker mode on and using the maximum output setting.

dia but are not in full cardiac arrest. There are four potential complications:

1. Induction of Ventricular Fibrillation. There is a possibility that VF may be induced when bradyarrhythmias are paced. This risk is, however, largely theoretical. Unlike epicardial electrodes, which easily induce VF, transcutaneous electrodes deliver a broad electrical charge to the myocardium as a whole. The current required to induce fibrillation increases with increased pulse durations; the long duration impulses from transcutaneous pacemakers,

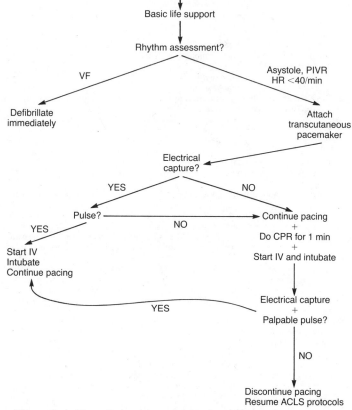

Figure 8–1. Flow diagram for use of transcutaneous pacing in cardiac arrest. PIVR = pulseless idioventricular rhythm; VF = ventricular fibrillation.

delivered at relatively low energy levels, pose little risk of VF induction.

2. Pain. A conscious patient will experience some muscle twitching and discomfort from transcutaneous pacemakers. The modern transcutaneous pacemaker minimizes pain because of long pulse durations, lower energy levels, a broad surface area for the impulse, and high-impedance electrode gel. Several studies have reported the discomfort as only "mild or moderate and easily tolerated."

3. Tissue Damage. Transcutaneous pacing appears safe for brief use (30–60 minutes) in humans. Other than some local skin erythema and first-degree burns, there have been few reports of direct tissue damage following transcutaneous pacing. Autopsies performed on people who were transcutaneously paced for 2 to 3 days revealed no evidence of pacer-induced myocardial damage. In animal models the energy level required to induce tissue damage from repeated direct countershocks has been 1000 times greater than the energy level required to pace the heart transcutaneously. Cardiac enzymes and serial electrocardiograms in animals paced for 30 minutes over their intrinsic rhythm displayed no evidence of ischemic injury or infarction, and when the dogs were sacrificed 3 days later there was no clinically significant myocardial damage observed.

4. Operator Injuries. The current that flows between the two pacing electrodes is of such low energy and relatively long duration that it poses little risk to the operator. In fact, one manufacturer recommends that manual chest compressions be continued during the first minute of transcutaneous pacing, in order to "prime the myocardium" to respond to the pacing impulses. In addition, chest compressions are recommended when electrical capture but not mechanical capture occurs. Operators who have given chest compressions while the pacemaker discharges its impulses report little more than a slight tingling to their hands. Whether or not this "priming of the myocardium" is a valid physiologic concept is unclear. The practice, however, confirms that the operators are at small risk during transcutaneous pacing.

A Perspective on Transcutaneous Pacing

The efficacy of transcutaneous pacing for patients in cardiac arrest from asystole has not yet been established, although case reports of rare successes continue to be published. There is, however, clearly a use for transcutaneous pacing for patients with symptomatic bradycardias that are unresponsive to atropine or adrenergic stimulants. In addition, transcutaneous pacing may prove to be most useful for those cardiac arrest patients who have asystole as the initial rhythm following a defibrillatory shock (secondary asystole, or post-defibrillation asystole), although, again, the evidence is largely anecdotal.

We do not recommend that transcutaneous pacemakers be purchased primarily for use on patients with asystole, because the evidence that now exists would not justify such a recommendation. However, if a transcutaneous pacemaker is to be purchased by an emergency room or a prehospital rescue unit for immediate use in patients with symptomatic bradycardias (of proven efficacy), the devices should also be tried on patients with primary or secondary asystole or PIVRs (of anecdotal efficacy).

Our strong recommendation is that if protocols do include transcutaneous pacing for certain cardiac arrest rhythms, the pacing must come early in the protocol. This means before, or simultaneous with, endotracheal intubation and intravenous medications.

If rescuers employ transcutaneous pacing only as a "last ditch" effort, failure is virtually assured.

TRANSVENOUS PACEMAKERS

In the cardiac arrest or emergency situation transcutaneous pacemakers are preferred initially. However, if they are not available, transvenous or transthoracic pacemakers may be tried.

Insertion of Temporary Transvenous Pacemakers

Percutaneous transvenous pacemakers should be inserted under fluoroscopic guidance by a skilled operator. In the cardiac arrest situation, emergency transvenous pacing is indicated when a hemodynamically unstable bradycardic rhythm or torsade de pointes occurs that is unresponsive to drug and fluid therapy. It is occasionally used in cases of ventricular asystole when a central line is already in place.

Equipment and Supplies: Prepackaged trays are commercially available.
1. Material for skin sterilization and sterile technique.
2. Equipment and supplies for central line placement, whichever site is chosen.
3. Introducer with obturator or 14-gauge needle.
4. Pacemaker wire and power source.

Procedure:
1. Follow the insertion instructions for whichever central line site is chosen: antecubital, subclavian, internal jugular, or femoral (least preferred). Instead of the introducing needle for the central catheter, the introducer for the pacemaker wire is used. Making a small (0.5–1 cm) skin incision with a No. 11 scalpel blade will facilitate insertion of the pacemaker introducing needle.
2. Estimate the distance from the insertion site to the right ventricle, to get a rough idea of when the pacemaker wire should be capturing. Distances are usually 45–50 cm for the antecubital and femoral routes, and 15–20 cm for the internal jugular and subclavian routes.
3. Note the direction of curvature of the tip of the pacemaker wire, and maintain orientation so that it curves toward the atrium as it is inserted.
4. Insert the pacemaker wire into the introducer and advance it toward the right ventricle. This is best done under fluoroscopic guidance. If fluoroscopy is not available, insert the wire one-half the estimated distance to the ventricle and attach it to the power source. Set the power source to high (5 milliamperes) at a rate of

70–80 beats per minute. Watch the electrocardiograph or monitor while advancing the wire. The wire is against the right ventricular wall when pacer spikes are seen in front of QRS complexes. Advance the wire another centimeter to make sure it is anchored in the right ventricular wall.

5. Reduce the power to the lowest amperage that allows continuous capture.

6. If successful, anchor the pacing wire securely with a skin suture and dress the wound. Arrange for insertion of a transvenous or permanent pacemaker as soon as possible.

7. If fluoroscopy was not available, obtain an immediate portable chest x-ray to determine the position of the pacemaker wire and to check for pneumothorax.

TRANSTHORACIC PACEMAKERS

Insertion of Temporary Transthoracic Pacemaker

This method of pacemaker insertion should be used almost exclusively as a last resort, because of the potential for complications such as cardiac laceration, coronary artery penetration, pericardial tamponade, hemothorax, and pneumothorax.

Equipment and Supplies: Prepackaged pacemaker trays are commercially available.

1. Material for skin sterilization and sterile technique.

2. Introducer with obturator or 18-gauge spinal needle.

3. Syringe, 5–10 ml.

4. Pacemaker wire and power source.

5. No. 11 scalpel blade with holder.

6. Skin suture (4-0 or larger) with cutting needle, needle holder, and scissors.

7. Tape, gauze sponges, and antibacterial ointment.

Procedure:

1. Sterilize the skin around the patient's xiphoid and maintain sterile technique.

2. Stop chest compression.

3. Locate the site of insertion just to the left and below the tip of patient's xiphoid and make a small (0.5 cm) skin incision with the No. 11 scalpel blade.

4. Insert the introducer needle through the skin incision at a 30–40° angle to the skin and advance the needle toward the patient's left shoulder.

5. Remove the obturator periodically to check for blood flow either spontaneously or with a syringe.

6. When blood flows freely, the ventricle has been entered. Remove the obturator and immediately occlude the hub with a thumb. Pass the entire pacing wire into the introducer, being

careful not to let go of the end of the wire. When the end of the wire reaches the hub, withdraw the wire and needle as a single unit until the introducer is outside the skin. While holding the pacing wire where it enters the skin, remove the introducing needle.

7. Connect the end of the pacer wire to the power source, making sure the terminals are inserted into the proper location.

8. Withdraw the pacing wire carefully until it meets resistance.

9. Turn the power source to high (5 milliamperes) at a rate of 70–80 per minute. Watch the ECG or monitor for signs of capture or pacemaker spike. Reduce power to the lowest amperage that still allows for pacing.

REFERENCES

1. Falk RH, Zoll PM, Zoll RH: Safety and efficacy of noninvasive cardiac pacing: a preliminary report. N Engl J Med 309:1166, 1983.
2. Olsen CM, Jastremski MS, Smith RW, et al: External cardiac pacing for out-of-hospital bradyasystolic arrest. Am J Emerg Med 3:129, 1985.
3. Zoll PM, Zoll RH, Falk RH, et al: External noninvasive temporary pacing: clinical trials. Circulation 71:937, 1985.
4. Dalsey WC, Syverud SA, Hedges JR: Emergency department use of transcutaneous pacing for cardiac arrests. Crit Care Med 13:399, 1985.
5. Falk RH, Jacobs L, Sinclair A, et al: External noninvasive cardiac pacing in out-of-hospital cardiac arrest. Crit Care Med 11:779, 1983.
6. Paris PM, Stewart RD, Kaplan RM, et al: Transcutaneous pacing for bradyasystolic cardiac arrests in prehospital care. Ann Emerg Med 14:320, 1985.
7. Syverud SA: Transcutaneous cardiac pacing. In Roberts JR, Hedges JR (eds): Clinical Procedures in Emergency Medicine. Philadelphia, WB Saunders, 1985, pp 201–206.
8. Syverud SA, Dalsey WC, Hedges JR, et al: Transcutaneous cardiac pacing: determination of myocardial injury in a canine model. Ann Emerg Med 12:261, 1983.
9. White JM, Nowak RM, Martin GB, et al: Immediate emergency department external cardiac pacing for prehospital bradyasystolic arrest. Ann Emerg Med 1985;14:298, 1985.
10. Hedges JR, Syverud SA, Dalsey WC: Development in transcutaneous and transthoracic pacing during bradyasystolic arrest. Ann Emerg Med 1984;13:822, 1984.
11. Wiegle A, White RD: Non-invasive pacing: a pre-hospital ALS alternative. J Emerg Med Services 10:35, 1985.

9

DRUGS USED IN RESUSCITATION

ANTIARRHYTHMICS

Lidocaine

Lidocaine is the drug of choice in the acute management of ventricular premature beats, ventricular tachycardia, and ventricular fibrillation. It should also be used to suppress ventricular irritability following successful electrical conversion of ventricular fibrillation or ventricular tachycardia. The prophylactic use of lidocaine is recommended in patients with a high probability of having an acute myocardial infarction.

> **Lidocaine Dosage:** *For cardiac arrest:* 1 mg/kg IV (or intratracheally, if an endotracheal tube is in place prior to an IV), then 0.5 mg/kg bolus every 5–10 minutes as necessary to a total of 3 mg/kg, followed by a 2–4 mg/min continuous infusion.
> *For other settings:* 1 mg/kg IV, followed by a continuous IV infusion of 2 mg/min. If ectopy persists, repeat 0.5 mg/kg boluses every 10 minutes and increase the infusion by 1 mg/min after each bolus to a maximum of 4 mg/min. A 4 mg/ml solution is prepared by adding 1 g of lidocaine to 250 ml D5W.

Cautions: Patients with congestive heart failure, severe liver disease, shock due to any cause, and age over 70 years should be given half the normal bolus dose and observed closely for signs of toxicity. However, in the presence of ventricular fibrillation, the initial bolus of 1 mg/kg is still recommended. The earliest signs of lidocaine toxicity are CNS related and can range from slurred speech, altered consciousness or behavior, or muscle twitchings to seizures or respiratory arrest. If lidocaine toxicity is suspected, the dosage must be reduced immediately and other antiarrhythmics, such as procainamide, instituted for persistent ectopy.

Procainamide

In ACLS, procainamide is used primarily to suppress ventricular premature beats and ventricular tachycardia when lidocaine is ineffective or contraindicated.

> **Procainamide Dosage:** 100 mg IV every 5 minutes until the arrhythmia is suppressed or 1 g has been administered, followed by a continuous infusion of 1–4 mg/min.
>
> A 2 mg/ml solution is prepared by adding 500 mg of procainamide to 250 ml D5W.

Cautions: Blood pressure and QRS interval must be monitored carefully. Hypotension or widening of the QRS interval by 50% of its original width is a sign of procainamide toxicity, and its administration must be temporarily discontinued. Since procainamide is excreted primarily in the urine, patients with renal failure should be given a lower maintenance dose. Patients requiring more than 3 mg/min infusion for over 24 hours should have blood levels monitored.

Bretylium

Bretylium is a quaternary ammonium compound useful in the treatment of ventricular fibrillation and ventricular tachycardia. Since it is no more effective than lidocaine, bretylium is currently the second drug of choice, after lidocaine, in the treatment of refractory or recurrent ventricular fibrillation or unstable ventricular tachycardia. It is the third drug of choice, after lidocaine and procainamide, in the treatment of hemodynamically stable ventricular tachycardia.

> **Bretylium Dosage:** *For VF or pulseless VT:* 5 mg/kg IV bolus, followed by defibrillation. If arrhythmia persists, increase the bolus to 10 mg/kg every 15–30 minutes to a maximum total dose of 30 mg/kg. Defibrillate after each bolus.
>
> *For persistent VT:* 5–10 mg/kg diluted to 50 ml with D5W and infused over 8–10 min, followed by a continuous infusion at a rate of 1–2 mg/min. A 2 mg/ml solution is prepared by adding 500 mg of bretylium to 250 ml D5W.

Cautions: Bretylium induces a chemical sympathectomy-like state by inhibiting norepinephrine release from adrenergic neurons. Thus, postural hypotension occurs regularly, and supine hypotension occasionally, following its administration. In addition, bretylium aggravates digitalis toxicity and must be used with caution in digitalized patients.

Atropine

Atropine is a parasympatholytic drug useful in the treatment of unstable bradycardias (presence of hypotension, chest pain, confusion, PVCs) and ventricular asystole. It accelerates the sinus rate and facilitates conduction at the AV node by its vagolytic action.

Atropine Dosage: For bradycardia: 0.5 mg IV boluses every 5 minutes until adequate response or a total dose of 2 mg is reached.

For asystole: 1.0 mg IV bolus, repeated in 5 minutes if needed. Atropine can also be given through an endotracheal tube if IV access is delayed.

Cautions: In the setting of acute MI, atropine can increase ventricular irritability. Also, if the heart rate is accelerated excessively, myocardial ischemia may be worsened and the area of infarction enlarged. Thus, bradycardia that is hemodynamically stable or asymptomatic should not be treated with atropine.

Verapamil

Verapamil is a calcium channel inhibitor that slows conduction through the AV node. It is used to convert PSVT (paroxysmal supraventricular tachycardia) with a narrow QRS complex to sinus rhythm in stable patients who are unresponsive to vagal maneuvers (e.g., carotid sinus massage). Unstable patients with PSVT may be given verapamil while emergency cardioversion is readied. In atrial flutter or fibrillation, verapamil can slow ventricular response but seldom will convert it to sinus rhythm.

Verapamil Dosage: 5 mg IV bolus, then 10 mg in 15–30 minutes if PSVT persists and there is no adverse reaction to the initial dose.

Cautions: Verapamil has vasodilating and negative inotropic effects that may cause hypotension and worsen left ventricular dysfunction. Thus, it is contraindicated in patients with congestive heart failure. Because of its action on the AV node, it should also not be used in patients with 2nd or 3rd degree AV block. Severe bradycardia may occur, especially in patients with sick sinus syndrome. Rapid ventricular response can occur in patients with accessory pathways, as seen in Wolff-Parkinson-White or Lown-Ganong-Levine syndrome. Calcium chloride, 0.5–1.0 g IV, can be given to attempt to reverse the adverse effects of verapamil.

Propranolol

Propranolol is a fast-acting beta-blocker useful in the treatment of hemodynamically significant SVT (supraventricular tachycardia). It is a fourth-line drug used to treat ventricular arrhythmias unresponsive to lidocaine, bretylium, and procainamide.

> ***Propranolol Dosage:*** 1–3 mg IV given slowly every 5 minutes up to a total dose of 0.1 mg/kg.

Cautions: Propranolol should be avoided in patients with heart failure, second- or third-degree AV block, or asthma, since beta-stimulation may be a critical factor for clinical stability.

ADRENERGIC AGONISTS

Isoproterenol

Isoproterenol is a pure beta-agonist useful in the temporary treatment of hemodynamically significant bradycardia that is resistant to atropine, until a pacemaker can be inserted.

> ***Isoproterenol Dosage:*** 2–20 mcg/min continuous IV infusion titrated to the desired heart rate response. A 2 mcg/ml solution is prepared by adding 1 mg of isoproterenol to 500 ml D5W.

Cautions: Isoproterenol stimulates potent chronotropic and inotropic responses that result in improved cardiac output at the expense of increased myocardial work. If the increase in myocardial perfusion does not compensate for the increased myocardial oxygen consumption, myocardial ischemia can worsen. In addition, isoproterenol causes peripheral vasodilatation that can result in severe hypotension if the increase in cardiac output is not sufficient. Isoproterenol can also cause and exacerbate arrhythmias.

Epinephrine

Epinephrine has both alpha- and beta-stimulating properties that improve both myocardial and cerebral blood flow as well as increase inotropy and coarsen ventricular fibrillation. It is used in the cardiac arrest setting for the management of ventricular fibrillation, ventricular asystole, and electromechanical dissociation. It is seldom used solely for its pressor effect, since more effective drugs are available (e.g., dopamine, norepinephrine).

> ***Epinephrine Dosage:*** 0.5–1.0 mg of a 1:10,000 solution given IV every 5 minutes as necessary.
> If intubation is completed prior to establishment of IV access, 1.0 mg of a 1:10,000 solution can be given intratracheally. The same dose can also be given intracardially, if a central line is not available and resuscitation is unsuccessful.

Cautions: Epinephrine does increase myocardial work and decrease renal perfusion, but these considerations are moot in the cardiac arrest setting.

Norepinephrine (Levophed)

Norepinephrine is a potent alpha-agonist that increases peripheral resistance by causing peripheral vasoconstriction. It is especially useful in the management of shock associated with low peripheral vascular resistance (e.g., septic shock). It is not effective in the treatment of hypovolemic shock.

> ***Norepinephrine Dosage:*** Start at 8 mcg/min continuous IV infusion given into a large vein via an infusion pump, and titrate to the desired blood pressure response. A 16 mcg/ml solution is prepared by adding 4 mg of norepinephrine to 250 ml D5W.

Cautions: Continuous intra-arterial pressure monitoring is recommended during the administration of norepinephrine, since auscultated blood pressures may be inaccurate because of vasoconstriction. Norepinephrine also increases myocardial work and may worsen myocardial ischemia. Extravasation of norepinephrine can cause severe ischemia and necrosis of local tissue. Phentolamine (an alpha-antagonist), 5–10 mg in 10–15 ml of saline solution, should be infiltrated liberally to the area of extravasation as soon as possible. Norepinephrine is contraindicated in patients using monoamine oxidase (MAO) inhibitors or tricyclic antidepressants, since severe hypertension may result.

Dopamine

Dopamine is a norepinephrine precursor that has variable beta- and alpha-adrenergic and dopaminergic effects, depending on the dose. At low levels (2–10 mcg/kg/min), the dopaminergic and beta-adrenergic effects dominate to produce increased cardiac output while dilating renal and mesenteric blood vessels. At moderate doses (10–20 mcg/kg/min), all three effects are present. At high doses (over 20–30 mcg/kg/min), the alpha-adrenergic effect predominates, and renal perfusion is no longer spared. Dopamine is the usual drug of choice in the treatment of nonhypovolemic shock.

> **Dopamine Dosage:** 2–20 mcg/kg/min continuous IV infusion, given via infusion pump, starting at the lower dose and titrating to the desired hemodynamic effect. A solution containing 800 mcg/ml is prepared by adding 200 mg of dopamine to 250 ml D5W.

Cautions: Hemodynamic monitoring is recommended whenever dopamine is used. Because dopamine is metabolized by monoamine oxidase, it must be used with caution and the dosage decreased in patients treated with MAO inhibitors. Since dopamine is inactivated by alkaline solutions, it should not be given in the same IV line with sodium bicarbonate. Like norepinephrine, extravasation of dopamine should be treated with infusion of phentolamine (5–10 mg in 10–15 ml saline solution) into the extravasation site.

Dobutamine

Dobutamine is a potent inotropic agent with primarily beta$_1$-receptor stimulating effects. It is useful in the short-term management of heart failure caused by decreased myocardial contractility. Dobutamine and nitroprusside have a synergistic effect when used concomitantly.

> **Dobutamine Dosage:** 2.5–20 mcg/kg/min continuous IV infusion, given via an infusion pump, starting at the lower dose and titrating to desired effect. A 500 mcg/ml solution is prepared by adding 250 mg to 500 ml D5W.

Cautions: Hemodynamic monitoring is recommended for optimal benefit when dobutamine is used. At doses over 20 mcg/kg/min, an increase in heart rate is commonly seen that may worsen ischemia. Dobutamine facilitates conduction through the AV node and can induce a rapid ventricular response in patients with inadequately treated atrial fibrillation. Dobutamine is contraindicated in patients with hypertrophic obstructive cardiomyopathy.

VASODILATING AGENTS

Nitroglycerin

Sublingual Route: When administered sublingually, nitroglycerin (NTG) is rapidly absorbed (1–2 min) and is highly effective in treating angina.

> **Nitroglycerin Dosage:** 0.4 mg (1/150 gr) sublingually every 5 minutes up to 3 tablets. Patients with suspected angina should seek immediate medical attention if pain is unrelieved after 3 tablets.

Cautions: Headache and orthostatic hypotension are common side effects of sublingual NTG. Thus, patients should be instructed to be seated or in a supine position while taking NTG. Transient supine hypotension can occasionally occur, especially in dehydrated patients, and is usually responsive to placement in the supine position with the legs elevated (Trendelenburg).

Dermal Route: Nitroglycerin ointment is absorbed rapidly and has a prolonged effect. It mainly causes peripheral venous dilatation (preload reduction), and it may be useful in the acute treatment of hypertension or cardiogenic shock until hemodynamic monitoring is available for the use of more potent drugs such as nitroprusside.

> **Nitroglycerin, Dermal Dosage:** ½–2 inches every 4–6 hours as needed.

Cautions: Nitroglycerin ointment can also cause headache and orthostatic hypotension. If symptoms are severe, the effect can be promptly relieved by wiping away the ointment.

Intravenous Route: Intravenous nitroglycerin is useful in the treatment of congestive heart failure and ischemic chest pain not relieved by sublingual NTG or morphine. NTG causes relaxation of vascular smooth muscle, especially of the venous system. Thus, peripheral venous capacitance increases, reducing venous return to the heart (preload), and peripheral vascular resistance decreases (afterload), resulting in reduced left ventricular filling pressures and improved cardiac output. Myocardial oxygen demand decreases while coronary perfusion increases, thus improving congestive heart failure and overall hemodynamic state. Nitroglycerin is preferred over nitroprusside in patients with congestive heart failure, since nitroglycerin-induced arterial vasodilatation wanes as left ventricular filling pressure decreases, so that coronary perfusion pressure is maintained. In contrast, nitroprusside-induced arterial dilatation is not affected by a reduction of filling pressure.

> ***Nitroglycerin, IV Dosage:*** 10 mcg/min continuous IV infusion via infusion pump, increasing by 5 mcg/min every 3–5 minutes until desired effect. Preparation of solution varies depending on the brand used. Follow the manufacturer's instructions.

Cautions: Hemodynamic monitoring should be used in patients with congestive heart failure. Side effects include hypotension and headache, as with the other routes of administration.

Nitroprusside

Nitroprusside is a direct arterial and venous vasodilator that improves cardiac output and relieves pulmonary edema by reducing both preload and afterload, similar to the hemodynamic effects of intravenous nitroglycerin. In addition, it is a potent hypotensive agent that is useful in the management of hypertensive crisis and dissecting aortic aneurysm with hypertension. The action of nitroprusside is almost immediate and ends when the infusion is stopped, allowing for close titration.

> ***Nitroprusside Dosage:*** 0.5–10 mcg/kg/min continuous IV infusion via an infusion pump, starting at the lowest dose and titrating to desired effect. A 200 mcg/ml solution is prepared by adding 50 mg of nitroprusside to 250 ml D5W. The container and tubing should be wrapped with aluminum foil, since nitroprusside will deteriorate with exposure to light.

Cautions: Hemodynamic monitoring is recommended whenever nitroprusside is used for congestive heart failure. Intra-arterial monitoring is recommended when nitroprusside is used for hypertensive crisis. Nitroprusside is metabolized to cyanide, which is then metabolized to thiocyanate in the liver. Metabolic acidosis is one of the earliest signs of cyanide toxicity and must be closely monitored. Serum thiocyanate levels should be monitored if nitroprusside is used for longer than 48 hours, especially in patients with renal insufficiency. Signs of thiocyanate toxicity are tinnitus, blurred vision, and alteration of mentation.

Nifedipine

Nifedipine is a calcium channel blocker useful in the treatment of angina, especially angina due to coronary artery spasm (e.g., Prinzmetal or ergonovine-induced). It is also useful in the acute treatment of hypertension.

> **Nifedipine Dosage:** *For angina:* 10 mg orally initially, increasing by 10-mg increments to a total of 30 mg over 4–6 hours. Maintenance dose is 10–30 mg, 3–4 times/day.
> *For hypertension:* 10 mg sublingually; may repeat as needed in 30–60 minutes.

Cautions: Blood pressure must be closely monitored after nifedipine administration, since excessive hypotension occasionally occurs. Peripheral edema due to arterial vasodilation may occur and must be differentiated from that due to congestive heart failure. Since nifedipine may increase the serum digoxin level, digoxin levels should be monitored in all patients taking that drug.

DIURETICS

Furosemide and Ethacrynic Acid

Furosemide (Lasix) and ethacrynic acid (Edecrin) are potent diuretics useful in the treatment of pulmonary and cerebral edema. Furosemide also causes direct venodilatation that further reduces left ventricular filling pressure (preload). This effect can be evident within 5 minutes after IV administration, whereas diuresis may be delayed for over 20 minutes.

> **Furosemide or Ethacrynic Acid Dosage:** 20–40 mg IV bolus; repeat at higher dose if not effective after 15 minutes.

Cautions: Electrolyte imbalance, especially hypokalemia, and excessive diuresis resulting in dehydration can occur following administration of a potent diuretic.

MISCELLANEOUS AGENTS

Digoxin

Digoxin is useful in slowing the ventricular response rate of patients with hemodynamically stable atrial fibrillation or flutter with a rapid ventricular rate. It is seldom used now for its inotropic properties, because of the availability of other safer and more effective inotropic agents.

Digoxin Dosage: 0.25–0.50 mg IV bolus, followed by 0.25 mg IV every 2 hours until conversion to sinus rhythm or until ventricular rate is less than 100/min.

Cautions: Digoxin and other digitalis preparations have a narrow therapeutic range that is decreased even further by hypokalemia or administration of calcium. Serum digoxin levels must be followed closely, particularly in patients with renal insufficiency or congestive heart failure. GI symptoms and arrhythmias, especially PVCs, junctional escape rhythms, and atrial tachycardia with block, are the most common manifestations of digoxin toxicity.

Morphine

Morphine is a narcotic analgesic useful in the treatment of chest pain associated with myocardial ischemia or infarction. It is also useful in the management of acute pulmonary edema, because of its direct venodilating effect that reduces venous return to the heart (preload), thereby decreasing pulmonary congestion.

Morphine Dosage: 2–5 mg IV every 5–30 minutes until desired effect.

Cautions: Morphine, like all narcotics, can cause hypotension and respiratory and cerebral depression. Naloxone, a narcotic antagonist, can be given at a dose of 0.2–0.8 mg (0.4 mg/ampule) IV to reverse the undesired effects of morphine.

Calcium

Calcium is no longer recommended in the management of cardiac arrest unless hypocalcemia or toxicity due to calcium channel blocking agents is present. It has not been shown to be effective in the treatment of asystole or EMD, and it may actually interfere with resuscitation efforts.

Calcium Dosage: 2 ml of a 10% solution of calcium chloride IV, repeated as needed in 15–30 minutes, OR 5–7 ml of calcium gluceptate OR 5–8 ml of calcium gluconate.

Sodium Bicarbonate

Bicarbonate is no longer routinely recommended in the management of cardiac arrest. Acid-base balance is most effectively achieved by providing adequate ventilation to correct respiratory acidosis and by converting arrhythmias to a perfusing rhythm. Bicarbonate does not appear to improve the resuscitation effort, and it may actually decrease chances of resuscitation. Bicarbonate produces a more harmful cellular environment by shifting the oxyhemoglobin dissociation curve leftward, reducing the release of oxygen to ischemic tissues, and by increasing the production of CO_2, which can depress myocardial function. Excessive use of bicarbonate can also cause hypernatremia, hyperosmolarity, and alkalosis, which can further depress myocardial and cerebral function. Thus, bicarbonate should not be used during the first 10 minutes of resuscitation. Thereafter, it should be used only if severe metabolic acidosis is present, as determined by arterial blood gas measurements or at the discretion of the team leader. There may be a role for bicarbonate following restoration of pulse when accumulated lactic acids begin to perfuse the body.

Sodium Bicarbonate Dosage: 1.0 mEq/kg IV, followed by 0.25–0.50 mEq/kg every 10–15 minutes as needed.

Amrinone

Amrinone is an inotropic and vasodilator agent useful in the treatment of heart failure. It is a nonadrenergic agent similar to dobutamine in its hemodynamic effects.

Amrinone Dosage: 0.75 mg/kg IV bolus given over 2–3 minutes, followed by a continuous IV infusion of 5–10 mcg/kg/min. A 1 mg/ml solution is prepared by adding 100 mg (one 20-ml ampule) to 100 ml normal saline or half normal saline.

Cautions: Hemodynamic monitoring is recommended for optimal benefit when amrinone is used. Because of its intropic effect, amrinone may worsen myocardial ischemia. It may cause thrombocytopenia.

10

ARRHYTHMIAS

MANAGEMENT

The management of specific arrhythmias associated with cardiac arrest follows this section. Since cardiac resuscitation is often electrocardiographically dynamic, with frequent changes in rhythms, other cardiac rhythms are included for the sake of completeness.

The management of cardiac arrest requires much to be done rapidly and simultaneously. A single person should assign tasks and direct therapy. Control rather than chaos can prevail only if a standard approach is used. The following approach and protocols are based on the American Heart Association's *Standards and Guidelines for Emergency Cardiac Care*, published in JAMA, June 6, 1986 (reprinted with permission of the publishers). These guidelines and protocols should not preclude flexibility in the management of cardiac arrhythmias.

Guidelines and Protocols

1. Confirm cardiac arrest—patient unconscious, with absent or agonal respirations and no pulse.

2. If cardiac arrest is witnessed, a precordial thump should be given.

3. Determine cardiac rhythm with "quick-look" paddles or cardiac electrodes if a defibrillatory monitor is present. We recommend that the few extra seconds be used to attach electrode leads, as the ECG signal is far more accurate with electrode leads compared with quick-look paddles. We have seen instances in which the tremulous hand of the defibrillator operator using quick-look paddles resulted in a false signal of ventricular fibrillation.

4. Defibrillatory shocks, if ventricular fibrillation is present, are the most important aspect of therapy and should be provided as soon as possible.

5. CPR should be initiated if shocks are unsuccessful or until a defibrillator is available. Establish an open airway and ventilate mouth-to-mouth or with a pocket mask or bag-valve-mask device. Supplement with 100% O_2 if possible. Verify effective ventilation by observing chest wall motion.

6. Establish an IV line. Use D5W unless hypovolemia as the cause of arrest is suspected. If at all possible, CPR should not be interrupted.

7. Intubate with an endotracheal tube (an esophageal obturator

airway should be used only if endotracheal intubation cannot be done), and check for bilateral and equal breath sounds. Each intubation attempt should take no more than 20 seconds.

8. Administer medications and/or additional defibrillatory shocks as prescribed under "Therapy" in the following sections on specific arrhythmias.

Additional Comments

1. *Tachyarrhythmias, bradyarrhythmias, AV block*, and *hypotension* (discussed in the following sections) should be treated vigorously during resuscitation and the immediate post-resuscitation period.

2. *Complications of CPR:* Numerous complications can result from CPR. These should be anticipated, especially if CPR is performed for a long time and/or is initiated by an untrained bystander. Complications include:

   a. Pneumothorax or hemothorax of the lung resulting from a fractured rib puncturing the lung or a vessel.
   b. Aspiration of stomach contents.
   c. Laceration of the liver or spleen, with internal bleeding.
   d. Contusion of the heart.
   e. Puncture of the coronary artery, or pneumothorax secondary to laceration of the lung, which may occur from intracardiac injection.

VENTRICULAR FIBRILLATION

Because of the importance of ventricular fibrillation, more information is included in this section, including discussion of refractory ventricular fibrillation.

Diagnosis

1. Ventricular fibrillation (VF) is the most frequently encountered rhythm in sudden cardiac death, seen in approximately 60% of all cases. Consciousness is lost within seconds. There is no pulse or blood pressure. Frequently collapse occurs without warning symptoms. In other cases, symptoms suggestive of myocardial infarction or ischemia may precede the collapse. Ventricular fibrillation may also result from hypoxia, electrolyte disorders, acidosis, and hypothermia. Ventricular fibrillation rarely, if ever, spontaneously changes to an organized rhythm. Defibrillatory shocks are required to stop (defibrillate) ventricular fibrillation.

2. *Defibrillatory shocks* are the most important aspect of therapy for VF, and the sooner they are given, the more likely they are to be successful.

3. *Identification of VF:* Rhythm is chaotic in appearance, with marked variation in amplitude frequency and morphology. There are no organized complexes. Rate is indeterminate, but frequency of defibrillations on the ECG is fast (>300/min). Ventricular fibrillation may be coarse, medium, or fine. This distinction is arbitrary, as VF does not consist of multiple rhythms; rather, the appearance of VF depends upon its duration (and probably the underlying condition of the heart). Initially, VF is coarse in appearance; as VF continues, the amplitude of deflection decreases such that within several minutes VF is "regular" in appearance; and as VF continues still longer, the amplitude becomes less and less. By 10–15 minutes, VF appears fine, and beyond 15–20 minutes it become asystole. The distinction between fine VF and asystole is difficult to determine precisely. Clinical studies have revealed that the probability of return to a perfusing rhythm after a countershock depends upon the amplitude of the VF waveform, as well as a variety of other factors.

4. *Mechanical Aspects of VF:* During VF, the contractile process in the myocardium is completely disorganized and uncoordinated. Effective contractions are lost, tissue perfusion is absent, and cellular death soon ensues. In the absence of CPR, blood flow through the coronary arteries is nonexistent. There is some dispute over whether coronary artery blood flow can occur during fibrillation even with the chest compressions of basic CPR. A number of clinical and laboratory studies suggest that the positive effects of CPR appear to be twofold: (1) a prolongation of the length of time that VF is present, and (2) an increase in the probability that the rhythm after defibrillation will be a perfusing one. This evidence implies that even though the heart is in fibrillation, some coronary blood flow must occur through the coronary arteries during CPR chest compression.

5. *Physiology of VF:* VF is a rhythm disorder that results from a disturbance of both automaticity (impulse formation) and impulse conduction (re-entry). Normally ventricular re-entrant tachy-arrhythmias are prevented by the refractory period of depolarized myocardium. During VF, however, the normal orderly depolarization sequence in the ventricles is completely lost. Several factors, most commonly ischemia, act both to shorten the heart's refractory period and to increase the conduction velocity. Self-perpetuating wavefronts of wandering depolarization can develop, but only if the heart has a certain size or "critical mass." The hearts of small mammals will fibrillate only while an electrical stimulus is applied. Fibrillation stops when the stimulus is withdrawn. Experiments with the fibrillating hearts of larger animals have demonstrated that surgical removal of pieces of the ventricles will stop the fibrillation once a critical mass of the heart no longer remains. Similarly, infusion of potassium chloride into one branch of the

left coronary artery will not stop fibrillation, but upon infusion into both branches, the fibrillation ceases.

6. VF can be confused with artifact, especially if quick-look paddles are used or if leads are not fully attached.

VENTRICULAR FIBRILLATION (VF)

Diagnostic Criteria	Causes
Irregular undulations of different shapes No distinct QRS complexes VF may be coarse, medium, or fine	Myocardial infarction, coronary artery disease, hypoxia, acidosis, electrolyte imbalance

The following criteria distinguish fine, medium, and coarse VF. Amplitude is measured peak-to-trough over at least a 3–6 second period. Asystole is defined as an average amplitude of 0–<1 mm. These criteria, while arbitrary, are clinically useful.

a. Coarse VF—average amplitude >7 mm:

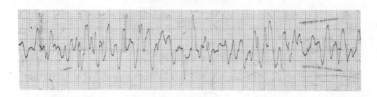

b. Medium VF—average amplitude 3–<7 mm:

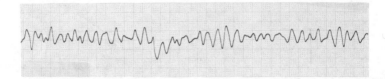

c. Fine VF—average amplitude 1–<3 mm:

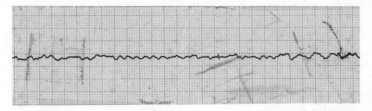

Therapy

1. The management for VF is outlined in Figure 10–1. The first step, confirming cardiac arrest, should be accomplished by seeing

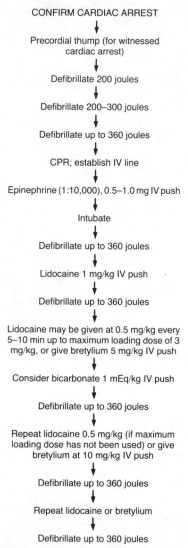

CONFIRM CARDIAC ARREST

↓

Precordial thump (for witnessed cardiac arrest)

↓

Defibrillate 200 joules

↓

Defibrillate 200–300 joules

↓

Defibrillate up to 360 joules

↓

CPR; establish IV line

↓

Epinephrine (1:10,000), 0.5–1.0 mg IV push

↓

Intubate

↓

Defibrillate up to 360 joules

↓

Lidocaine 1 mg/kg IV push

↓

Defibrillate up to 360 joules

↓

Lidocaine may be given at 0.5 mg/kg every 5–10 min up to maximum loading dose of 3 mg/kg, or give bretylium 5 mg/kg IV push

↓

Consider bicarbonate 1 mEq/kg IV push

↓

Defibrillate up to 360 joules

↓

Repeat lidocaine 0.5 mg/kg (if maximum loading dose has not been used) or give bretylium at 10 mg/kg IV push

↓

Defibrillate up to 360 joules

↓

Repeat lidocaine or bretylium

↓

Defibrillate up to 360 joules

Figure 10–1. Management of ventricular fibrillation.

that the patient is unconscious and unresponsive and that no carotid pulse is present.

2. Witnessed cardiac arrest should have a precordial thump.

3. Rapid defibrillation is the most important aspect of therapy and should precede CPR, IV medications, and intubation. If a

defibrillator is not immediately available, CPR should be performed until one is.

4. The rhythm should be checked after each shock. Pulse should be checked if an organized rhythm is present. The initial three shocks should be given as rapidly as possible, assuming VF persists.

5. Epinephrine (0.5–1.0 mg IV) should be given every 5 minutes for persistent VF.

6. Assuming ventilation is possible without intubation, intubation should be delayed until after the initial 3 shocks and epinephrine have been given.

7. Bicarbonate, 1 mEq/kg IV push, is considered after 5 shocks, epinephrine, and antiarrhythmics have been tried. The value of bicarbonate is questionable, and evidence suggests that it may be harmful. If severe acidosis is suspected (for example, an unwitnessed cardiac arrest with a prolonged resuscitation and difficulty in ventilation), the use of bicarbonate may be helpful. Bicarbonate, if used, may be repeated every 10 minutes, 0.5 mEq/kg IV push.

8. If defibrillation is successful, lidocaine infusion (1–4 mg/min IV) should be started. If lidocaine has not previously been given, a 1 mg/kg IV bolus should be given before the infusion.

Refractory VF

Unfortunately, a significant number of people in VF, treated as outlined above, may either remain in VF or develop recurrent VF. In recurrent VF, the countershocks successfully defibrillate the myocardium, but the heart soon refibrillates. The two interventions most beneficial in this situation are endotracheal intubation with administration of 100% O_2, and intravenous administration of antifibrillatory medications. Intubation and antifibrillatory medications are discussed elsewhere in this book. In patients who refibrillate, one must consider what the rhythm was during the brief period of non-VF rhythms. The therapeutic approaches may be different.

When faced with refractory or recurrent VF, and defibrillation, intubation, and intravenous antifibrillatory agents are unsuccessful, the following should be considered as possible causes (listed in order of recommended consideration):

1. **Acidosis.** Consider improper placement of the endotracheal tube, pneumothorax, pericardial tamponade, and the need for bicarbonate.

2. **Alkalosis.** Alkalosis can cause or perpetuate ventricular dysrhythmias. It shifts the oxyhemoglobin dissociation curve to the left, which prevents adequate delivery of oxygen to the tissues. Alkalosis can be caused by excessively rapid ventilation. The rate of ventilation should be reduced, and sodium bicarbonate should be withheld.

3. **Excessive Parasympathetic Stimulation.** There are occasionally patients in whom the sequence is: (a) VF, (b) defibrillation to

a transiently normal sinus rhythm, bradycardia, or asystole, and (c) refibrillation to VF. In this situation, excessive parasympathetic stimulation may be present. Intravenous atropine (0.5 mg every 5 minutes to a total of 2 mg) may speed up any underlying supra-ventricular rhythm and prevent recurrence of the VF. Overdrive pacing with one of the newly available transcutaneous pacemakers (see Chapter 8) may stabilize the rhythm and prevent return of VF.

4. Excessive Catecholamine Stimulation. If, however, a patient in VF is defibrillated to a rapid sinus tachycardia and yet that rhythm becomes unstable and the patient refibrillates, the problem may be excessive catecholamines. Additional epinephrine should be withheld and intravenous propranolol (1–3 mg every 5 minutes to a total of 0.1 mg/kg) be considered. Alternatively, verapamil has been used successfully in this situation. The patient with recurrent VF during a resuscitation attempt may then respond to repeat defibrillatory shocks when loaded with propranolol.

5. Hypokalemia. There is some clinical evidence that sudden death and lethal arrhythmias in otherwise normal hypertensive patients may have been triggered by diuretic-induced hypokalemia. Potassium supplementation is absent in many patients on diuretics, and 25–50% of these patients develop hypokalemia. Potassium depletion enhances automaticity, alters myocardial conduction velocity, and can cause a wide spectrum of atrial and ventricular dysrhythmias. Faced with an unstable and hypokalemic patient who is suffering recurrent VF with only brief periods of a stable rhythm between defibrillations, aggressive potassium replacement should be considered: 10 mEq of potassium chloride diluted in 50 ml of D5W given over 30 minutes; repeat every 30 minutes until serum potassium measures between 4.0 and 5.0 mEq/L. Iatrogenic hyperkalemia can be prevented by continuous ECG monitoring.

6. Hypomagnesemia. This problem, often combined with hypokalemia, is frequently observed in malnourished patients, in alcoholics, and in patients on diuretics. Malignant rhythm disturbances, including VF, can occur with low serum magnesium levels, particularly if hypokalemia is simultaneously present. Hypomagnesemia can be corrected relatively rapidly: 1–2 g of magnesium sulfate (2–4 ml of a 50% solution) diluted in 50 ml of D5W and given IV over 15 minutes. Once this and other electrolyte abnormalities have been corrected, recurrent acute episodes of VF may disappear or additional attempts at defibrillation may be successful.

VENTRICULAR FLUTTER

Ventricular flutter is a transitional rhythm between ventricular tachycardia and ventricular fibrillation, and is usually present for a very brief time. The management is the same as that of ventricular fibrillation.

VENTRICULAR FLUTTER

Diagnostic Criteria	Causes
Rate: 150–300 *Rhythm:* regular *P wave:* none *P:QRS:* none *QRS:* no distinct QRS complexes; rhythm is a transitional stage between ventricular tachycardia and ventricular fibrillation	Same as for ventricular fibrillation

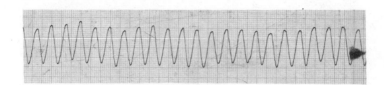

Ventricular flutter

VENTRICULAR TACHYCARDIA

Diagnosis

1. Ventricular tachycardia (VT) is an arrhythmia that is extremely serious and potentially fatal because of associated fall in cardiac output, increased myocardial O_2 demand, decreased coronary flow, and resultant deterioration of vital signs. Ventricular tachycardia, depending upon the underlying condition of the patient and the condition of the heart, may be tolerated for variable periods of time. In many intances, VT is tolerated for only seconds before consciousness is lost and cardiac arrest ensues. In other situations, VT can be tolerated for minutes or even hours.

2. Ventricular tachycardia may be self-terminating or it may persist (usually over seconds to minutes), degenerating into ventricular fibrillation. Frequently in cardiac arrest, VT occurs for a few beats and immediately becomes VF.

3. The effect of VT on vital signs is variable, the spectrum being immediate cardiac arrest (no pulse or blood pressure) to normal vital signs with VT tolerated for hours. Usually, VT leads to signs and symptoms (fall in blood pressure, angina, dizziness, shortness of breath) requiring immediate therapy.

4. VT can be confused with wide QRS tachycardia (for example, paroxysmal atrial tachycardia [PAT] or sinus tachycardia with aberrant conduction). The most helpful electrocardiographic clue to distinguish VT from wide QRS tachycardia is ventriculoatrial dissociation (no relation of P and QRS waves). The presence of ventriculoatrial dissociation indicates VT.

5. *Identification:* Three or more successful ectopic ventricular beats occurring at a rate of over 100 per minute (usually 140–200/min). QRS complexes are >0.12 second, with features of PVCs (see p. 138). VT that continues is termed sustained VT.

VENTRICULAR TACHYCARDIA (VT)

Diagnostic Criteria	Causes
Rhythm: slightly irregular *P wave:* may be noted as atria continue to discharge *P:QRS:* no relationship *QRS:* >0.12 second	Myocardial infarction, coronary artery disease, hypoxia, acidosis

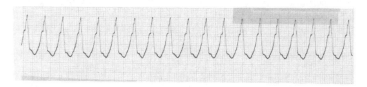

Ventricular tachycardia

Therapy

1. The hemodynamic status of the patient determines the therapy and aggressiveness of the therapy (see Fig. 10–2).

2. VT patients in cardiac arrest (no pulse) should be treated exactly the same as patients in ventricular fibrillation.

3. Patients with a pulse should be treated as outlined in Figure 10–2. Therapy is based on the patient's condition, i.e., whether stable or unstable. Unstable refers to the presence of chest pain, shortness of breath, hypotension (<90 mm Hg systolic), congestive heart failure, ischemia, or infarction.

4. In the absence of hypotension, pulmonary edema, or unconsciousness, a precordial thump may be tried prior to cardioversion.

5. In the patient in an urgent condition—unconsciousness, hypotension, or pulmonary edma—unsynchronized shocks may be used to avoid delay of synchronization.

6. If lidocaine, procainamide, or bretylium converts VT, a maintenance infusion should be started. If cardioversion occurs prior to administration of lidocaine, a 1 mg/kg IV bolus should be given followed by a 1–4 mg/min IV maintenance infusion. If hypotension, pulmonary edema, or unconsciousness is present, use lidocaine if cardioversion alone is unsuccessful, followed by bretylium. In all other patients, the recommended order of therapy is lidocaine, procainamide, and then bretylium.

7. Persistent VT that is not responsive to the protocol in Figure 10–2 may respond to propranolol, 0.5–1.0 mg/min IV, up to 5 mg.

8. Sedation, if necessary prior to cardioversion, can be accom-

plished with diazepam (Valium) given in 2–5 mg increments IV until the patient becomes drowsy (have patient count backward from 100; when numbers are missed, the level of sedation is probably acceptable).

Alternatively, methohexital sodium (Brevital) may be used (500 mg in 250 ml D5W, administered by rapid microdrip infusion). Drowsiness frequently begins within 25 ml. Sufficient sedation is indicated by lack of response to eyelid stimulation. At this point, stop the infusion and proceed with cardioversion. Valium and Brevital can lead to respiratory depression. Therefore, it may be necessary to artificially ventilate the patient.

9. Torsade de pointes is a specific type of ventricular tachycardia that requires different treatment. The term torsade de pointes means "turning of the points" and refers to the shifting and alternating orientation of the QRS complex.

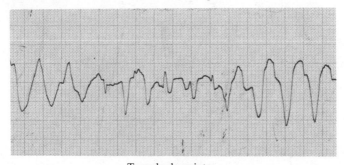

Torsade de pointes

Torsade de pointes appears similar to polymorphic ventricular tachycardia (VT with two or more ectopic sites predominating), and may be impossible to distinguish in the prehospital setting. It is associated with a long QT interval in the complexes preceding the tachycardia. Torsade de pointes does not respond to the usual VT therapy. In some patients, isoproterenol has been successful, but electrical overdrive pacing is the treatment of choice. Procainamide is contraindicated.

ASYSTOLE

Diagnosis

1. Asystole is the end result of ventricular fibrillation or other rhythms. On rare occasions asystole may be the result of increased parasympathetic tone.

2. The prognosis, even with successful resuscitation, is extremely poor.

3. Rarely, ventricular fibrillation may masquerade as asystole (owing to a vector of VF). Therefore, when asystole is encountered it should be verified with another ECG lead or repositioning of the electrodes.

4. Always check calibration cables, electrodes, cable paddle switch, and low battery indicator to confirm that asystole is not artifactual.

5. *Identification:* Absent electrical activity or amplitude of ECG signal < 1 mm, sometimes with occasional agonal contractions.

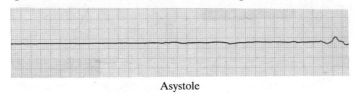

Asystole

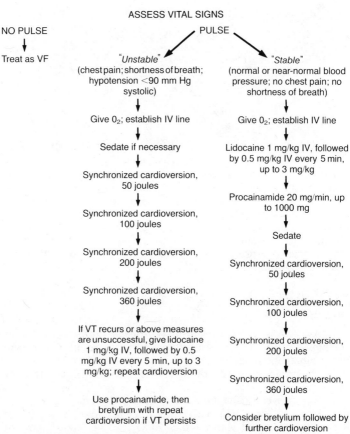

Figure 10–2. Management of ventricular tachycardia.

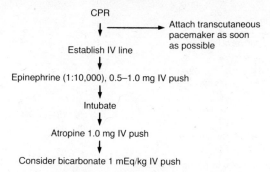

Figure 10–3. Management of asystole.

Therapy

1. The management of asystole is shown in Figure 10–3. Asystole should be confirmed in two leads or with repositioning of chest electrodes.

2. Note that the protocol differs in sequencing from the American Heart Association's guidelines. The AHA guidelines recommend that early pacing be considered after an IV line has been established, and after intubation, epinephrine, and atropine have been tried. We recommend transcutaneous pacing (if available) as soon as possible. This does not mean that IV placement, intubation, or administration of drugs should be delayed. Instead, pacing and other procedures should proceed simultaneously.

3. If it is unclear whether fine VF or asystole is present, provide defibrillatory shocks as indicated in the VF protocol.

4. Epinephrine, 0.5–1.0 mg IV, should be repeated every 5 minutes.

5. Atropine, 1.0 mg IV, may be repeated in 5 minutes.

6. The value of bicarbonate is questionable, and evidence suggests that it may be harmful. Bicarbonate, if used, should initially be given at a dosage of 1 mEq/kg IV push and may be repeated every 10 minutes at a dosage of 0.5 mEq/kg IV push.

ELECTROMECHANICAL DISSOCIATION

Diagnosis

1. Electromechanical dissociation (EMD) is usually associated with severe myocardial damage and carries a grave prognosis.

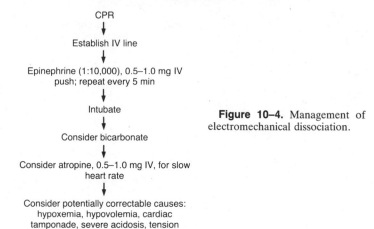

CPR
↓
Establish IV line
↓
Epinephrine (1:10,000), 0.5–1.0 mg IV
push; repeat every 5 min
↓
Intubate
↓
Consider bicarbonate
↓
Consider atropine, 0.5–1.0 mg IV, for slow
heart rate
↓
Consider potentially correctable causes:
hypoxemia, hypovolemia, cardiac
tamponade, severe acidosis, tension
pneumothorax, pulmonary embolism

Figure 10–4. Management of electromechanical dissociation.

2. *Identification:* The term EMD refers to organized electrical activity (sinus, ventricular, or nodal) without effective muscular contraction. In other words, an organized complex is seen on the monitor, but there is no pulse or blood pressure.

3. EMD usually is associated with underlying heart disease and frequently occurs in the setting of massive myocardial infarction. It may also be the result of hypoxemia, hypovolemia, severe acidosis, pericardial tamponade, tension pneumothorax, or pulmonary embolism.

Therapy

1. The management of EMD is similar to that of asystole (see Fig. 10–4).

2. Epinephrine, 0.5–1.0 mg IV, should be repeated every 5 minutes.

3. The use of bicarbonate is questionable, and there is evidence that it may be harmful. Bicarbonate, if used, should initially be given at a dose of 1 mEq/kg IV and then repeated every 10 minutes (0.5 mEq/kg IV).

4. Always consider potentially correctable causes of EMD: hypoxemia, hypovolemia, cardiac tamponade, severe acidosis, tension pneumothorax, pulmonary embolism.

IDIOVENTRICULAR RHYTHM

Diagnosis

1. Idioventricular rhythm is a specific type of EMD. Rates range from 20–40/min and are regular. P waves are usually not present. QRS is widened and bizarre appearing.

IDIOVENTRICULAR RHYTHM

Diagnostic Criteria	Causes

Rate: 20–40/min
Rhythm: regular
P wave: usually not present
P:QRS: no relationship
QRS: >0.11 sec; wide,
  bizarre-appearing
	Myocardial infarction,
	  hypoxia, acidosis

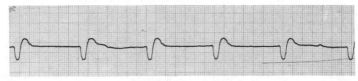

Idioventricular rhythm

Therapy

1. Therapy is the same as for EMD (see p. 126).
2. Atropine, 1.0 mg IV, may be tried in an attempt to speed the heart rate and perhaps achieve a palpable pulse.

PAROXYSMAL SUPRAVENTRICULAR TACHYCARDIA (PSVT)

Diagnosis

1. A common arrhythmia seen both in patients with normal hearts and in those with abnormal hearts.
2. Also commonly referred to as paroxysmal atrial tachycardia (PAT).

PAROXYSMAL SUPRAVENTRICULAR TACHYCARDIA (PSVT)

Diagnostic Criteria	Causes
Rate: 150–250/min *Rhythm:* regular; usually starts and stops abruptly *P wave:* upright in I, II, aVF; may be buried in preceding T wave *P:QRS:* 1:1	Often seen in individuals with no evidence of heart disease; may be precipitated by sympathetic nervous system stimulation, emotion, fatigue, caffeine, or alcohol; less common causes are cardiac surgery, thyrotoxicosis, and pulmonary embolus

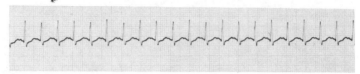

Paroxysmal supraventricular tachycardia (PSVT)

Therapy

The decision to treat with physical maneuvers, pharmacologic therapy, or cardioversion is based upon the patient's condition (see Fig. 10–5).

Physical Maneuvers

Patients who are stable may be treated with maneuvers to transiently increase vagal tone. These include carotid sinus massage

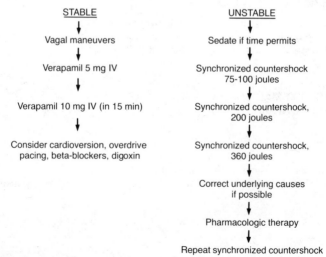

Figure 10–5. Management of paroxysmal supraventricular tachycardia.

(CSM), Valsalva maneuver, gagging, lying with head down and legs elevated while taking deep inspirations, or facial immersion in iced water for 30 seconds. CSM and facial immersion should not be used in patients with atherosclerotic heart disease. CSM should not be performed if a carotid bruit is present. Start CSM on right side; if unsuccessful, try left side. *Never* massage both carotids simultaneously. All of the above maneuvers should occur with the patient monitored and an IV in place, with atropine (0.5 mg) available. If maneuvers to increase vagal tone are unsuccessful, they should be repeated after drug therapy, as Valsalva or CSM frequently potentiates pharmacologic effects.

Pharmacologic Therapy

Stable patients who do not respond to vagal maneuvers should receive verapamil.

1. Dosage of verapamil is 5 mg IV given over 1 minute (3 minutes in elderly). It may be repeated in 15 minutes if necessary at a dose of 10 mg IV.

2. Contraindications to verapamil include hypotension and congestive heart failure.

3. The most commonly seen complication following verapamil is hypotension. This is more likely to occur in patients on chronic beta-blocker therapy. Hypotension can often be reversed with calcium chloride, 0.5–1.0 g IV, given slowly.

4. Patients who fail to respond to verapamil should be treated in the hospital. Options for treatment include elective cardioversion, beta-blockers, overdrive pacing, digitalis, and sedation.

Cardioversion

Patients who are unstable must be treated promptly with synchronized cardioversion. Unstable conditions include hypotension with chest pain or shortness of breath, congestive heart failure, decreased level of consciousness, and PSVT occurring with associated myocardial infarction.

1. Cardioversion should be done with synchronized countershock, 75–100 joules initially. Subsequent synchronized shocks, if needed, should be at 200 and 360 joules.

2. If the patient is conscious, sedate with diazepam, 2–5 mg increments IV until drowsiness occurs, or with Brevital (see p. 123).

3. Contraindications to countershock include suspected digitalis toxicity and recurrent PSVT after conversion to sinus rhythm. If electric cardioversion is initially successful and PSVT recurs, other therapies should be used prior to additional shocks.

ATRIAL FLUTTER

Diagnosis

1. Atrial flutter should be strongly suspected in patients with a regular ventricular rate of 150/min.

2. Ventricular rhythm is usually regular, with a 2:1 AV conduction ratio; "grouped beating" with alternating 2:1 and 4:1 conduction may occur.

3. Atrial flutter is frequently confused with sinus tachycardia, PAT with block, junctional tachycardia, or ventricular tachycardia (particularly when aberrant AV conduction is present).

4. Carotid sinus massage often brings out flutter waves by increasing AV block in a stepwise fashion, e.g., from 2:1 to 4:1.

5. Atrial flutter is usually seen in patients with underlying heart disease.

6. Episodes are often triggered by stress, trauma, infection, hypoxia, hyperthyroidism, and drugs (e.g., quinidine or Pronestyl in treatment of atrial fibrillation, as well as epinephrine and ephedrine); occasionally by alcohol withdrawal and ketoacidosis; and rarely by digitalis toxicity.

ATRIAL FLUTTER

Diagnostic Criteria	Causes
Rate: variable, depending on degree of atrioventricular block *Rhythm:* atrial is regular at >300/min; ventricular rate and rhythm rate may or may not be regular, depending on degree of block *P wave:* flutter waves, commonly described as sawtooth pattern *P:QRS:* usually 2 or more P flutter waves to 1 QRS; commonly 2:1, 3:1 or 4:1, but can be variable	Coronary artery disease, mitral valve disease, pulmonary embolism, after cardiac surgery

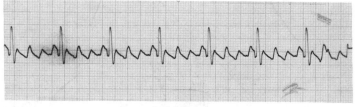

Atrial flutter

Therapy

1. Treat underlying disorder: heart failure, hyperthyroidism, infection, and so forth.

2. Synchronized countershock is the treatment of choice and should be done emergently in patients with hemodynamic compromise. Start with 25 joules and increase by 50-joule increments if unsuccessful. Digitalis toxicity is a contraindication in all but desperate circumstances. Recent food ingestion is a relative contraindication in nonemergent situations.

3. Digoxin is an alternative therapy. Digoxin increases AV block and ventricular contractility and may convert atrial flutter to atrial fibrillation with a controlled ventricular rate. Cardioversion can still be used if the patient's condition worsens, but generally this should be done before >1.25 mg digoxin has been given. If the fully digitalized patient is being cardioverted, it is desirable to discontinue digoxin for 1 to 2 days. If cardioversion must be done immediately, start with 5–10 joules, increasing to 100 joules in small increments. If postshock ventricular premature beats occur, give 50–100 mg lidocaine IV before subsequent shocks.

4. Verapamil is an alternative therapy and will usually slow the ventricular rate even if conversion does not occur.

5. Propranolol can be used to slow the heart rate in urgent circumstances unless contraindicated (e.g., by severe congestive heart failure, asthma, AV block). Dosage is 0.5–1.0 mg/min IV up to 5 mg with BP and ECG monitoring, followed by oral maintenance (20 to 60 mg orally every 6 hours).

6. For patients with recurring paroxysmal atrial flutter, maintenance digoxin (0.125–0.375 mg orally daily) may help prevent episodes or control ventricular rate during episodes. Quinidine is useful in preventing recurrences when digoxin alone is ineffective. Usual dosage: quinidine sulfate, 300–400 mg orally every 6 hours, or quinidine gluconate, 324–486 mg (1–1½ tablets) orally every 8 hours. (See digoxin-quinidine interaction under Atrial Fibrillation, p. 134.)

7. Right atrial pacing is useful in recurrent resistant flutter or when digitalis toxicity is suspected. Administration of 10 milliamperes at a rate faster than the flutter rate is often successful, but pacing rates up to 600/min may be required.

ATRIAL FIBRILLATION

Diagnosis

1. Atrial fibrillation occurs in the presence of myocardial disease with atrial involvement, especially rheumatic mitral disease, hypertension, arteriosclerotic cardiovascular disease, chronic lung disease, and hyperthyroidism. Occasionally it occurs without associated heart disease.

2. Precipitating factors include sympathetic or strong parasympathetic activity (nausea and vomiting, heavy alcohol use, hypogly-

cemia, postsurgical stress), myocardial infarction, and hypokalemia.

ATRIAL FIBRILLATION

Diagnostic Criteria	Causes
Rate: variable; atria are contracting at rate >350, but only a fraction of the signals fire the atrioventricular node; atrial fibrillation is considered fast if the ventricular rate is >100/min, and slow if ventricular rate is less than 60/min	Congestive heart failure, thyrotoxicosis, mitral stenosis, pulmonary embolus, coronary artery disease, cor pulmonale, restrictive pericarditis, after cardiac surgery
P wave: no discernible P wave; usually there is an irregular undulating baseline.	
P:QRS: QRS complexes occur at irregularly irregular intervals	

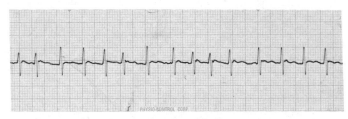

Rapid atrial fibrillation

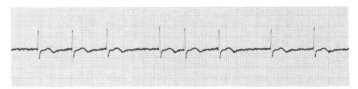

Atrial fibrillation

Therapy

1. Treat underlying disease: hyperthyroidism, hypokalemia, infection.

2. In the absence of hypotension or severe heart failure requiring emergency cardioversion, digoxin is the drug of choice for control of ventricular rate. It may be given orally or intravenously, as follows:

   a. PO: 0.75–1.0 mg followed by 0.25–0.5 mg every 6 hours for up to 24–48 hours (usual digitalizing dose: 2–2.5 mg).

   b. IV: 0.75 mg followed by 0.25 mg every 2–6 hours × 1–3 (usual digitalizing dose: 1–1.5 mg).

3. Maintenance dosage (0.125–0.375 mg daily) is initiated when heart rate is controlled (70–80/min at rest).

4. Patients with Wolff-Parkinson-White syndrome with widened QRS complex and rapid ventricular rate should be treated with propranolol or cardioversion rather than digitalis. Digitalis may increase conduction through the anomalous pathway and increase the ventricular rate.

5. Digoxin is contraindicated in suspected digitalis toxicity (sometimes identified by accelerated junctional rhythm in patient taking a digitalis drug) or in the presence of hypokalemia.

6. If digoxin is not effective in controlling ventricular rate, or if the clinical situation requires more urgent therapy, verapamil is usually successful in slowing the ventricular rate. Initial dose is 5 mg IV given over 1 minute (3 minutes in elderly). It may be repeated in 15 minutes at a dosage of 10 mg IV (see p. 129).

7. In paroxysmal atrial fibrillation without hemodynamic compromise, sedation may be helpful. Verapamil or digoxin often controls ventricular rate, and spontaneous cardioversion frequently occurs. If hemodynamic status worsens, no further digitalis should be given, and cardioversion with countershock should be attempted.

Emergency Cardioversion

Cardioversion may be indicated if hypotension, angina, or pulmonary edema results from acute onset of atrial fibrillation (frequently seen with acute myocardial infarction).

Sedation (diazepam IV, 2–5 mg increments) is indicated if the patient is conscious.

Digitalis toxicity is a contraindication to cardioversion, because high levels of digitalis potentiate post-cardioversion arrhythmias. If 1.25 mg or less digoxin has been used in an unsuccessful attempt to control ventricular rate, the risk of cardioversion is acceptable in urgent circumstances (see Atrial Flutter Therapy, p. 131).

Hypokalemia and hypoxia should be corrected prior to cardioversion.

Use synchronized countershock: Start with 50 joules and increase progressively to 360 joules. Post-cardioversion arrhythmias are more common at higher levels of energy.

Elective Cardioversion

Cardioversion may be performed electively if atrial fibrillation is not associated with significant symptoms or with heart failure. Young patients with mild myocardial disease, atrial fibrillation of recent onset, and minimal left atrial enlargement are most likely to maintain sinus rhythm. Synchronized countershock (generally preferred) or "medical" cardioversion with digoxin and quinidine can be used. Anticoagulation treatment with warfarin sodium (Coumadin) for 2 weeks prior to cardioversion is desirable in order to minimize the possibility of systemic emboli (up to 3% incidence). Quinidine may be started before synchronized countershock and continued after emergency or elective cardioversion to help maintain sinus rhythm (usual dosage: 300–400 mg quinidine sulfate orally every 6 hours, or quinidine gluconate, 324–486 mg [1–1½ tabs] orally every 8 hours).

Ventricular rate is controlled with digoxin; digoxin is then held for 24 hours before elective cardioversion.

Recent studies indicate that therapeutic doses of quinidine increase serum digoxin levels significantly (average twofold increase). Clinical effects of digoxin appear to increase as well. Accordingly, daily digoxin dosage probably should be halved when quinidine is started, and the patient followed to reassess digoxin effect at the lower rate.

BRADYCARDIA AND AV BLOCK

Diagnosis

SINUS BRADYCARDIA

Diagnostic Criteria	Causes
Rate: less than 60/min *Rhythm:* regular *P wave:* upright in I, II, aVF *P:QRS:* 1:1	May be physiologic, as in a well-trained athlete, or secondary to drugs (propranolol) or to sinus node diseases

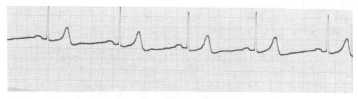

Sinus bradycardia

FIRST-DEGREE ATRIOVENTRICULAR BLOCK

Diagnostic Criteria	Causes
Rate: 60–100/min *Rhythm:* regular *P wave:* normal *P:QRS:* 1:1; PR interval is >0.20 sec	Coronary artery disease, digoxin, rheumatic fever, congenital conditions

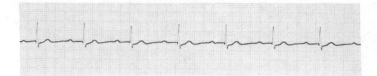

First-degree atrioventricular block

SECOND-DEGREE ATRIOVENTRICULAR BLOCK, MOBITZ TYPE I (WENCKEBACH)

Diagnostic Criteria	Causes
Rate: atrial rate is greater than ventricular rate *Rhythm:* atrial rhythm is regular; ventricular rhythm is irregular *P wave:* normal *P:QRS:* PR interval becomes progressively lengthened until a QRS is dropped; PP interval remains constant	Myocardial infarction, rheumatic fever, digitalis toxicity

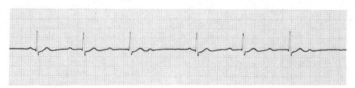

Second-degree atrioventricular block, Mobitz Type I (Wenckebach)

SECOND-DEGREE ATRIOVENTRICULAR BLOCK, MOBITZ TYPE II

Diagnostic Criteria	Causes
Rate: atrial rate is greater than ventricular rate *Rhythm:* atrial rate is regular; ventricular rate may be regular or irregular *P wave:* normal; PR interval is normal, and QRS usually shows bundle branch block *P:QRS:* ratio may be 2:1, 3:1, 4:1, or 3:2; ratio may vary over time; ratios of 2:1 are difficult to distinguish from Mobitz Type I; if in doubt, treat as Mobitz Type II	Myocardial infarction, digitalis toxicity

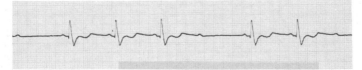

Second-degree atrioventricular block, Mobitz Type II

THIRD-DEGREE ATRIOVENTRICULAR BLOCK, COMPLETE HEART BLOCK

Diagnostic Criteria	Causes
Rate: atrial rate is greater than ventricular rate *Rhythm:* atrial rate is 60–100/min; ventricular rate is 40–60/min if junctional escape beats occur; ventricular rate is 20–40/min if ventricular rate escape beats occur *P wave:* normal *P:QRS:* no relationship; atria and ventricles are independently contracting *QRS:* normal if junction escape beats occur; >0.11 sec if ventricular escape beats occur	Coronary heart disease, myocardial infarction, myocarditis, drug toxicity (digitalis, procainamide, quinidine, verapamil)

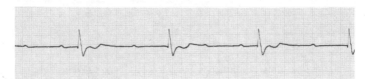

Third-degree atrioventricular block, complete heart block

Therapy

1. The management of bradycardia and AV block is determined by the condition of the patient. If the patient has a slow heart rate and is hemodynamically unstable (shows evidence of hypertension, altered mental status, chest pain, dyspnea), treatment is indicated (see Fig. 10–6).

2. Patients with sinus bradycardia, junctional bradycardia, 1° AV block or 2° AV block (Mobitz Type I) and who are hemodynamically stable (no hypotension or associated symptoms) may be observed.

3. Patients with 2° AV block (Mobitz Type II) or 3° AV block and who are hemodynamically stable should receive a transvenous pacemaker as soon as possible.

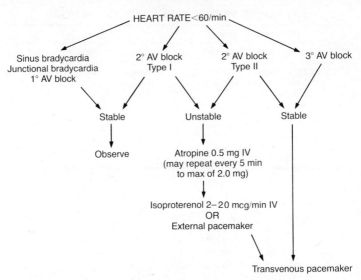

Figure 10–6. Management of bradycardia and A-V block.

4. For treatment of unstable bradycardia, regardless of the etiology, atropine is the drug of choice. Dosage of atropine is 0.5 mg IV, repeated as necessary every 5 minutes up to 2.0 mg. (Doses <0.5 mg are contraindicated because of occasional paradoxical slowing of the heart.)

5. If atropine is not effective, continued therapy with isoproterenol or external transcutaneous pacing is indicated. Dosage of isoproterenol (1 mg in 500 ml D5W = 2 mcg/ml) is 2–20 mcg/min IV. Isoproterenol and transcutaneous pacing are temporizing therapies, and arrangements should be made for insertion of a transvenous pacemaker.

PREMATURE VENTRICULAR CONTRACTIONS

Diagnosis

1. PVCs on routine ECG are frequently associated with significant heart disease: arteriosclerotic or hypertensive heart disease, cardiomyopathy, and acute rheumatic fever. However, PVCs occur in many persons who have no cardiac disease. PVCs are also seen in chronic respiratory disease, hypoxia, and infections (scarlet fever, diphtheria); with use of sympathomimetic drugs (epinephrine, isoproterenol, amphetamines, tricyclic antidepressants); in visceral reflexes with increased vagal tone; in anxiety, exercise, hypokalemia, and hypocalcemia; and with use of caffeine, tobacco, alcohol, and cardiac drugs (digitalis, quinidine, procainamide).

PREMATURE VENTRICULAR CONTRACTION (PVC)

Diagnostic Criteria	Causes
Rate: variable, depending on frequency of PVCs *Rhythm:* irregular *P wave:* no P wave association with PVC *P:QRS:* none *QRS:* >0.11 sec; PVCs may be unifocal or multifocal, and may be isolated or occur in a fixed relationship to the normal QRS	Coronary artery disease, myocardial infarction, hypoxia, acidosis, hypokalemia, stimulant drugs

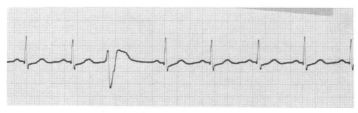

Premature ventricular contraction (PVC)

Differentiation of PVCs from supraventricular beats with aberrant conduction is often troublesome, but certain characteristics allow the distinction to be made (see Table 10–1).

Therapy

1. The approach to the patient with PVCs is outlined in Table 10–2 and Figure 10–7.

2. PVCs seen in patients without suspected acute MI may usually be observed with an effort made to treat the underlying cause (e.g., hypoxia).

3. PVCs (regardless of frequency or nature) should be vigorously treated if an acute infarction is suspected. Always consider correctable causes of PVCs. These include bradycardia (always treat bradycardia before treating PVCs), abnormalities of serum potassium, increased serum level of digitalis, and drugs (e.g., excessive beta-blockers).

   a. Initial treatment should be with lidocaine, 1 mg/kg IV push. If PVCs are not suppressed, repeat lidocaine at a dosage of 0.5 mg/kg IV push. Lidocaine (0.5 mg/kg IV push) should be repeated every 5 minutes (up to a total of 3 mg/kg) until PVCs are suppressed. Once PVCs are abolished, a lidocaine drip should be started (2–4 mg/min).

   b. If lidocaine is unsuccessful, procainamide and bretylium,

Table 10–1. DIFFERENTIAL CHARACTERISTICS OF PVCs AND ABERRANTLY CONDUCTED BEATS

Premature Ventricular Contraction	Aberrant Conduction
1. Fusion beats (combined normal contraction and PVC)	1. Preceding abnormal P wave
2. Left "rabbit ear" taller than right in V_1	2. Right "rabbit ear" taller than left in V_1
3. QS or rS complex in V_6	3. Triphasic contour in V_1 (rsR^1) and V_6 (QRS)
4. Initial vector usually different from normally conducted QRS	4. Initial vector same as that of normally conducted beats
5. R on T phenomenon	5. R on T rare (AV refractory period is usually long enough to prevent conduction at time of T wave)
6. Post-extrasystolic pause, fully compensatory	6. Short returning cycle; a normal beat at a short interval after an anomalous beat favors aberration, as temporary inhibition of AV conduction is not likely
7. PVC suggested if QRS ≥ 0.14 sec	7. Aberrant conduction suggested if QRS ≤ 0.12 sec

Table 10–2. MANAGEMENT OF PVCs

Condition	PVCs	Therapy
Suspected acute MI	PVCs	Suppressive therapy
	No PVCs	Consider prophylactic lidocaine
Chronic cardiac disease OR	<6 PVCs/min	Observe
Other disease	<6 PVCs/min R on T Multifocal Couplets Runs of VT	Treat underlying cause if possible Consider suppressive therapy with lidocaine

Need for suppressive therapy

↓

Lidocaine 1 mg/kg

↓

If PVCs not suppressed, repeat lidocaine 0.5 mg/kg every 5 min until no ventricular ectopy or up to 3 mg/kg given

↓

If not suppressed, give procainamide 20 mg/min, until no ventricular ectopy or up to 1000 mg given

↓

If not suppressed, give bretylium 5–10 mg/kg over 10 min

Once PVCs are suppressed, begin an infusion at the following doses:

After lidocaine 1 mg/kg: lidocaine drip, 2 mg/min

After lidocaine 1–2 mg/kg: lidocaine drip, 3 mg/min

After lidocaine 2–3 mg/kg: lidocaine drip, 4 mg/min

After procainamide: procainamide drip, 1–4 mg/min (check blood level)

After bretylium: bretylium drip, 2 mg/min

Figure 10–7. Suppressive therapy for premature ventricular contractions.

respectively, may be tried (see Fig. 10–7). If these are unsuccessful, overdrive pacing should be considered.

4. Patients with acute myocardial infarction (or a high likelihood of MI) without PVCs should be considered for prophylactic therapy with lidocaine. Evidence suggests that prophylactic lidocaine is beneficial in reducing the incidence of ventricular fibrillation even when PVCs are not present. Dosage is 1 mg/kg IV, followed in 10 minutes by 0.5 mg/kg IV and another 0.5 mg/kg IV in 10 minutes (loading dose, 2 mg/kg), followed by IV infusion of 2 mg/min. Local guidelines should be followed.

REFERENCES

1. Standards and guidelines for cardiopulmonary resuscitation (CPR) and emergency cardiac care (ECC). JAMA 255:2905, 1986.
2. Stewart RB, Bardy GH, Green L: Wide complex tachycardia: misdiagnosis and outcome after emergent therapy. Ann Intern Med 104:766, 1986.
3. DeSilva RA, Hennekens CH, Lown B, et al: Lidocaine prophylaxis in acute myocardial infarction: an evaluation of randomized trials. Lancet 2:855, 1981.
4. Koster RW, Dunning AJ: Intramuscular lidocaine for prevention of lethal arrhythmias in the prehospital phase of acute myocardial infarction. N Engl J Med 313:1105, 1985.
5. Carruth JE, Silverman ME: Ventricular fibrillation complicating acute myocardial infarction: reasons against the routine use of lidocaine. Am Heart J 104:545, 1982.

6. Dunn HM, McComb JM, Kinney CD, et al: Prophylactic lidocaine in the early phase of suspected myocardial infarction. Am Heart J *110*:353, 1985.

7. Morganroth J: Premature ventricular complexes: diagnosis and indications for therapy. JAMA *252*:673, 1984.

8. Olson DW, Thompson BM, Darin JC, et al: A randomized comparison study of bretylium tosylate and lidocaine in resuscitation of patients from out-of-hospital ventricular fibrillation in a paramedic system. Ann Emerg Med *13*:807, 1984.

9. Haynes RE, Chinn TL, Copass MK, et al: Comparison of bretylium tosylates and lidocaine in management of out of hospital ventricular fibrillation: a randomized clinical trial. Am J Cardiol *48*:353, 1981.

10. Myerburg JR, Estes D, Zaman L, et al: Outcome of resuscitation from bradyar-rhythmic or asystolic prehospital cardiac arrest. J Am Coll Cardiol *4*:1118, 1984.

11. Stueven HA, Tonsfeldt DJ, Thompson BM, et al: Atropine in asystole: human studies. Ann Emerg Med *13*:815, 1984.

12. Koster RW, Dunning AJ: Intramuscular lidocaine for prevention of lethal arrhythmias in the prehospital phase of acute myocardial infarction. N Engl J Med *313*:1105, 1985.

13. Stewart RB, Bardy GH, Greene L: Wide complex tachycardia: misdiagnosis and outcome after emergent therapy. Ann Intern Med 1986; *104*:766, 1986.

11

ACID-BASE BALANCE

INTRODUCTION

The subject of acid-base balance and the use of buffers in the setting of cardiac arrest has undergone controversy and change over the last several years. This chapter will discuss the areas of controversy and use the present knowledge base to derive some general conclusions about the evaluation and treatment of acid-base abnormalities in the setting of a cardiac arrest.

The Importance of Ventilation

Patients who suffer cardiac arrest develop serious acid-base abnormalities. Both metabolic and respiratory components come into play to determine the acid-base balance. A hypothetical diagram of these abnormalities is presented in Figure 11–1. During the down-time, when no CPR is administered, both metabolic and respiratory acidosis develop. Lactic acids accumulate from anaerobic metabolism, and carbon dioxide builds up and is unable to be excreted through the lungs. Once cardiopulmonary resuscitation (CPR) begins, the situation is only slightly improved. Closed-chest cardiac massage provides less than 30% of normal cardiac output. Even though ventilation is much improved, tissue hypoperfusion continues and lactate acidemia worsens. Adequate ventilation is an important function of CPR. It not only supplies oxygen to the pulmonary vasculature but also allows the excretion of carbon dioxide. Studies have demonstrated that endotracheal intubation and ventilation with high-flow oxygen is the ventilatory treatment of choice for patients in cardiac arrest. If equipment or personne are not available to accomplish endotracheal intubation, other methods may be used. These include mouth-to-mouth respiration, pocket-face-mask ventilation, or bag-valve-mask ventilation. However, the patient should be intubated as soon as practical during the course of treatment for the cardiac arrest.

The Arterial-Venous CO_2 Gap

Once adequate ventilation has been achieved, the most common acid-base abnormality encountered reflects a mixed pattern. As tissue hypoperfusion continues with closed-chest massage, lactate accumulates and a gradually worsening metabolic acidosis is seen both in the arterial and venous systems. The respiratory component

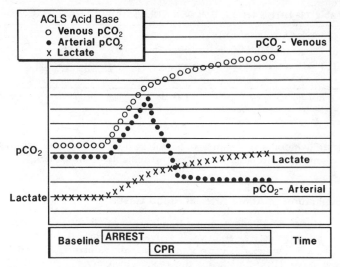

Figure 11–1. Hypothetical changes in venous and arterial pCO_2 and lactate levels during cardiac arrest. (ACLS = advanced cardiac life support.)

of acid-base balance, however, characteristically shows a divergent pattern of CO_2 levels in the arterial and venous systems (Fig. 11–1). Arterial P_{CO_2} is frequently normal or low, reflecting hyperventilation unless there is underlying pulmonary disease (pulmonary embolus, aspiration pneumonia, etc.). In contrast, venous blood shows marked hypercarbia and acidemia. If circulation is restored, this arterial-venous P_{CO_2} gap immediately closes. In order for the CO_2 to be excreted, the circulatory system must pick it up from the tissues and return it to the right side of the heart. The CO_2 must then be pumped into the pulmonary arteries with chest compressions and perfuse the lung tissue.

In the setting of a cardiac arrest and closed-chest massage, tissue perfusion—including lung perfusion—is marginal at best. In addition, the venous circulatory system may be ineffective in producing adequate venous return to the heart. Change in the intrathoracic pressure produced by chest compression is thought to impede venous return in the lower half of the body, where valves do not prevent retrograde blood flow through the inferior vena cava. Thus, because of the poor tissue perfusion and inefficient circulatory system, CO_2 as well as lactate accumulates in the venous system. This is thought to reflect a similar accumulation of CO_2 and lactate in the myocardium and other tissues. At the same time that CO_2 is accumulating in the venous system, the arterial blood may show an abnormal or low P_{CO_2}. Thus, the pH obtained in

Table 11–1. THE THREE GOLDEN RULES OF ACID-BASE BALANCE

I. Change ⇵ pCO_2 = change ⇵ pH 0.08 unit

II. Change ⇵ pH 0.15 unit = base change ⇵ 10 mEq/L

III. Total bicarbonate deficit = base deficit (mEq/L) × $\dfrac{\text{patient weight (kg)}}{4}$

(From the textbook of Advanced Cardiac Life Support of the American Heart Association.)

arterial blood gas samples may not be reflective of the acidosis present in the venous system and presumably in the tissues.

Evaluation of Acute Arterial Blood Gases

Arterial blood gases should be obtained in all patients suffering a cardiac arrest, as soon as it is feasible. When the results are obtained, the arterial Po_2 should be evaluated first. If the patient is hypoxic (Po_2 <80 torr), the oxygen delivery system must be reevaluated. Is the endotracheal tube correctly placed? Is supplemental oxygen being given? Are breath sounds adequate on both sides, with good respiratory expansion? If the oxygen delivery system is working properly, is there a primary pulmonary problem (e.g., pulmonary embolus, pneumonia) that must be addressed? Arterial hypoxia and hypercarbia in an arrest situation are poor prognostic indicators for successful resuscitation. Normal or near-normal arterial blood gases, however, are not predictive of successful resuscitation and should not be used as prognostic guidelines indicating that adequate CPR is being performed.

Following the evaluation of Po_2, one should evaluate the Pco_2 and acid-base status. A low Pco_2 (<35 torr) implies hyperventilation and an arterial respiratory alkalemia. A high Pco_2 (>35 torr) implies hypoventilation and an arterial respiratory acidemia. The contribution of the arterial Pco_2 determination to the overall acid-base abnormality can be determined by using approximations advocated by the American Heart Association, commonly referred to as the Golden Rules of acid-base balance (Table 11–1).

The overall acid-base status, however, depends upon other factors, such as venous and tissue CO_2 levels. Thus, while calculation of the extent of the metabolic acidosis is useful, treatment with sodium bicarbonate depends upon balancing the potential beneficial and harmful effects of therapy.

Because arterial pH and Pco_2 may not always be reflective of the acid-base imbalance in the venous system, it may also be useful to obtain a venous pH and Pco_2 in patients suffering from cardiac arrest. A comparison of the venous and arterial systems may give the physician better guidance on whether to treat the acidosis.

THE BICARBONATE THERAPY CONTROVERSY

Acidosis in Cardiac Arrest

Is acidosis bad for patients in cardiac arrest? The effect of acid-base abnormalities on myocardial function is unclear. The acid-base regulation of a myocardial cell is a complex function of both P_{CO_2} and bicarbonate and is not readily predicted from the extracellular pH.

Nevertheless, the majority of experimental studies indicate that acidosis suppresses myocardial contractility, lowers the fibrillation threshold, and attenuates the pressor response of catecholamines (Table 11-2). On the other hand, one can question the relevance of some of these observations for patients in cardiac arrest whose hearts are not contracting. What may be a more critical question is whether patients in ventricular fibrillation can be defibrillated. Studies have shown that arterial pH has little effect on defibrillation thresholds in animal models of fibrillatory arrest. Few outcome studies in humans have been done. However, one study showed that hypoxia, acidosis, and prolonged down-time were associated with unsuccessful defibrillation. Other studies in experimental animals failed to demonstrate the utility of pH as a predictor of successful resuscitation. Thus, overall there is experimental evidence that acidosis depresses myocardial function and attenuates the pressor response of catecholamines.

Buffer Treatment in Cardiac Arrest

If acidosis is bad for myocardial function, will treatment with buffers help? Two early animal studies demonstrated that when sodium bicarbonate was added to epinephrine in the treatment of animal models of cardiac arrest, resuscitation and 24-hour survival of the animals improved. Based on these data and empirical observations, bicarbonate treatment had become a mainstay of Advanced Cardiac Life Support therapy for acidosis in a cardiac arrest. Recent studies, however, have brought to light possible adverse effects of bicarbonate therapy. Patients receiving bicarbonate treatment for cardiac arrest were often found to be hyperosmolar and alkalotic, factors that were associated with unsuccessful outcome. Alkalosis also causes a shift of the oxygen hemoglobin dissociation curve to the left, making it more difficult to provide adequate tissue oxygenation.

When bicarbonate is administered to a patient with metabolic acidosis, it combines with the hydrogen ion to form carbonic acid. Carbonic acid is then dissociated to CO_2 and H_2O. Studies in the animal models and humans show that the administration of bicarbonate in the setting of cardiac arrest raises the arterial P_{CO_2} level.

Table 11–2. CASE EXAMPLE TO ILLUSTRATE THE THREE GOLDEN RULES OF ACID-BASE PROBLEMS

Case Example

A 60-year-old male who weighs 70 kg suffers a cardiac arrest. Arterial blood gas studies reveal:

$$pH = 7.10$$
$$P_{O_2} = 100 \text{ torr}$$
$$P_{CO_2} = 32 \text{ torr}$$

The P_{O_2} value of 100 torr indicates that the arterial system is getting adequate oxygen. However, the arterial P_{CO_2} of 32 torr indicates mild hyperventilation and a respiratory alkalosis. How much of the acid-base abnormality in the arterial blood (pH = 7.10) is determined by the respiratory component?

Normal P_{CO_2}	40 torr
Measured P_{CO_2}	−32 torr
Change from normal	8 torr

Application of Rules to Case Example

Golden Rule #1 lets us estimate how many pH units this value of 8 torr would represent. The rule states that 10 torr P_{CO_2} change = 0.08 pH change. A simple proportion lets us determine the pH change from 8 torr:

$$\frac{10 \text{ torr } P_{CO_2}}{8 \text{ torr } P_{CO_2}} = \frac{0.08 \text{ pH change}}{x}$$

$$x = 0.06 \text{ pH change due to respiratory alkalosis}$$

We now need to determine the metabolic component of the acid-base abnormality, which is calculated as follows:

Normal pH	7.40
pH change due to arterial respiratory alkalosis	+0.06
Calculated pH including arterial respiratory component	7.46
Measured pH from ABGs	−7.10
Metabolic component of acid-base abnormality	0.36 pH unit

How can we translate the metabolic pH unit change into a bicarbonate deficit?

Golden Rule #2 relates pH change to bicarbonate deficit. Once again, a proportion allows us to determine the base deficit:

$$\frac{0.15 \text{ pH}}{0.36 \text{ pH}} = \frac{10 \text{ mEq/L}}{x}$$

$$x = 24 \text{ mEq/L base deficit}$$

Golden Rule #3 allows us to translate the base deficit into the amount of bicarbonate needed based on the patient's weight:

$$\text{total bicarbonate deficit} = \text{base deficit} \times \frac{\text{weight (kg)}}{4}$$

$$= 24 \text{ mEq/L} \times \frac{(70 \text{ kg})}{4}$$

$$= 420 \text{ mEq bicarbonate}$$

Thus, this patient would need approximately 420 mEq of sodium bicarbonate to completely correct the metabolic acidemia.

The formation of CO_2 is helpful to the overall acid load of the body only if the CO_2 can be excreted in the lungs. As discussed above, excretion of CO_2 is already a problem because of the poor lung perfusion and circulation obtained with closed-chest massage. In addition, there is some concern that the increased P_{CO_2} obtained by the administration of bicarbonate may be harmful. Cellular membranes are generally more permeable to CO_2 than to bicarbonate. Thus, it is possible that intracellular acidosis could be worsened by the administration of bicarbonate and the increase in P_{CO_2}. Indeed, one experimental protocol showed an initial decrease in myocardial contractility after the intracoronary administration of bicarbonate in an animal preparation. Another study of bicarbonate administration in an animal model of lactic acidosis demonstrated that after bicarbonate was administered, blood pressure and cardiac index both significantly decreased, while lactate production increased. These changes may have been the result of increased intracellular acidosis due to the rise in CO_2.

CSF Acidosis

Another area of critical concern regarding the elevation of CO_2 following administration of bicarbonate is central nervous system acidosis. It has been observed that cerebral spinal fluid (CSF) pH does not necessarily reflect the blood pH in metabolic acidosis. However, CSF pH is closely correlated with blood pH states of respiratory acidemia. The explanation is thought to be that bicarbonate and some organic acids do not readily cross the blood-brain barrier but CO_2 does. Indeed, in an experimental animal model of cardiac arrest and bicarbonate treatment, CSF pH during CPR did not change as the blood pH became more acidotic. However, when bicarbonate was administered, CSF P_{CO_2} increased and CSF pH decreased while the blood pH increased. The paradoxical CSF acidosis is thought to be a reflection of the increased P_{CO_2} obtained after the administration of bicarbonate and its subsequent diffusion into the central nervous system.

A Note of Caution:

The clinical significance of these animal studies has yet to be determined. However, a note of caution about the possible adverse effect of bicarbonate therapy is in order. Good clinical outcome studies need to be done to determine the role of bicarbonate therapy in the treatment of patients in cardiac arrest. In addition, other buffers, such as tromethamine, are being investigated to determine if they can correct the acidosis without potential adverse effects. It is also prudent to remember that the root cause of the acid-base abnormalities seen in patients suffering cardiac arrest is the poor perfusion obtained in many patients undergoing CPR. If techniques can be developed that improve perfusion, problems from acidosis and its treatment are less likely to be significant.

CLINICAL RECOMMENDATIONS

Where does this leave the clinician trying to treat acid-base abnormalities of a patient in cardiac arrest? Each patient must be treated individually, with the physician balancing the possible helpful and harmful effects of each treatment given. There are some conclusions that can be gained from the data presented:

1. Hyperventilation seems to be the most effective method of attempting to correct acid-base abnormalities. In hyperventilating the patient and lowering Pco_2, the overall acid load for the patient is decreased.

2. It is important to remember that arterial blood gases may not reflect the acid-base status of the venous system or tissues. Obtaining venous as well as arterial pH and Pco_2 samples may aid in the overall evaluation of the acid-base status.

3. Patients who suffer cardiac arrest in which hyperkalemia may be a factor will benefit from bicarbonate treatment. Alkalinizing agents will decrease extracellular potassium and may be an important factor in the treatment of dysrhythmias, including ventricular fibrillation. Thus, in patients in whom hyperkalemia may be a factor, an initial dose of 1 mEq/kg of sodium bicarbonate should be used, followed by full replacement doses calculated by the ACLS Golden Rules.

4. Bicarbonate should not be routinely administered as a first-line drug. In other patients suffering from cardiac arrest, after 10 minutes in the treatment of the arrest victim, the clinician should consider whether treatment with sodium bicarbonate is indicated. The clinician must decide whether the potential benefits of treating the acidosis outweigh the potential adverse affects associated with increased Pco_2 levels. If bicarbonate treatment is decided upon, an initial dose of 1 mEq/kg should be used. Subsequent doses may be determined by the results of blood gas determinations. If these are unavailable, one-half the initial dose may be repeated every 10 minutes as needed.

12

CEREBRAL RESUSCITATION*

INTRODUCTION

Until recently, the incidence, severity, and correct therapeutic approach to neurologic damage following cardiac arrest remained largely unknown. It appears that, even in the best emergency medical systems, only 30–40% of patients who are resuscitated from out-of-hospital cardiac arrest will survive hospital discharge with intact neurologic function. The brain must never be forgotten—once a person has regained a perfusing rhythm following cardiac arrest, cerebral resuscitation must begin. Current investigative efforts, both laboratory and clinical, have focused on the pathophysiology of postischemic brain damage, and on the development of effective brain resuscitation techniques and therapies. This chapter reviews the pathophysiology of damage that occurs to the brain during and especially after cardiac arrest as it is presently understood, and discusses currently accepted and potentially promising therapies for improving neurologic recovery.

Neurologic outcome following cardiac arrest is determined by factors occurring before and during the cardiac arrest as well as after the return of circulation. Cardiac arrest, resulting in cessation of blood flow to the brain, creates *"global brain ischemia."* This ischemic insult can be divided into the following four components:

1. *Pre-arrest hypoxia time:* the duration of severe hypotension, hypoxemia, anemia, or other compromise of brain perfusion occurring immediately before the actual cardiac arrest.

2. *Arrest time* (also referred to as "time from collapse to CPR," or "down-time"): the duration of pulselessness without CPR.

3. *CPR time:* the time from the initiation of CPR until the restoration of a pulse (also referred to as "resuscitation time").

4. *Post-resuscitation hypoxia time:* the duration of hypotension, hypoxemia, anemia, or other compromise of brain perfusion that occurs immediately after restoration of spontaneous arterial pulsations.

After reperfusion of the brain, additional brain-damaging processes occur. These processes produce the *"post-resuscitation syndrome,"* or *"post-ischemic encephalopathy."*

---

*This chapter is adapted, with permission, from Abramson N, Safar P: Cerebral resuscitation. *In* Rosen P, Baker FJ II, Braen GR, et al: Emergency Medicine Concepts and Clinical Practice, 2nd ed. St. Louis, CV Mosby, 1987.

RELEVANT (AND IMPORTANT) PATHOPHYSIOLOGY

Brain Vulnerability. The brain is the organ of the body most vulnerable to ischemic insults, because of its high metabolic rate, oxygen comsumption, and blood flow requirements. Within 1 minute of total brain ischemia, brain ATP concentration decreases by 90%. There is a selective vulnerability of various brain areas, with the higher neuraxis functions—such as consciousness, intellect, personality, memory, and coordination—being the most commonly compromised neurologic functions following recovery from cardiac arrest.

Flow Thresholds. Neuronal synaptic transmission continues until cerebral blood flow falls below 35% of normal. At this level, the EEG becomes silent and functional ability is compromised, even though ions are still pumped across cell membranes. If cerebral blood flow falls to between 20 and 35% of normal, transmembrane ion pumping ceases, but cellular viability seems to be maintained. When cerebral blood flow falls below the "critical threshold" of 20% of normal, neuronal viability is compromised. Thus, the flow threshold for membrane failure is less than 20% of normal cerebral blood flow, and the flow threshold for functional failure is less than 35% of normal cerebral blood flow. The longer any of these compromised levels of perfusion exist, the more likely that cellular dysfunction or death will occur.

Ischemic Penumbra. Reperfusion following global brain ischemia does not produce a homogeneous diminution of blood flow. Rather, there are scattered areas of very low flow usually surrounded by better perfused areas, e.g., multifocal microinfarcts. Thus, there will be some cells that die during or after the ischemic insult, whereas other cells, either because they are less vulnerable to ischemia or because they receive higher blood flow during reperfusion, regain cellular function. Between these two extremes is the "ischemic penumbra," an area where cells have lost function but are still viable. The therapeutic efforts discussed in this chapter are directed primarily toward the preservation of these cells.

Reperfusion Injury. The very act of resuscitation can injure the brain through the damaging processes of the "post-resuscitation syndrome." This syndrome has several pathophysiologic phases:

1. *Hyperemic phase.* In this initial transient phase, perfusion is greater than normal, but unevenly distributed. It is unclear whether this increased flow actually perfuses the microcirculation.

2. *Hypoperfusion ("no-reflow") phase.* After 15–30 minutes of hyperemia, cellular edema begins to develop, along with clotting, red cell sludging, and platelet aggregation. Vasospasm develops, and cerebral blood flow deteriorates markedly. This hypoperfusion varies in severity throughout the brain and may last for 18–24

hours. Several physiologic mechanisms have been proposed to explain this "no-reflow" phenomenon, including increased intracranial pressure, cerebral vasoconstriction, decreased red blood cell deformability, platelet aggregation, pericapillary cellular edema, and abnormal calcium ion fluxes. The potential to reverse several of these abnormalities has therapeutic implications, and has recently captured the attention of investigators and clinicians.

3. *Recovery phase.* Following the hypoperfusion phase, regional cerebral blood flow may either improve, leading to functional recovery; remain low, leading to permanent coma; or continue to decline, resulting in brain death.

The Role of Calcium and Iron in Ischemia-Induced Cell Death. Current research for effective brain resuscitation therapies has focused on the role of calcium and iron in ischemia-induced cell death. Controversy surrounds these questions because it is unclear whether the pathophysiologic features observed with calcium and iron are the critical triggering mechanisms for ischemia-induced tissue injury or are merely epiphenomena that accompany the process of cell death.

Calcium Ion Fluxes. When cerebral blood flow falls below 20% of normal, a cellular influx of calcium ion is triggered. This intracellular calcium overload is thought to precipitate vasospasm, uncoupling of oxidative phosphorylation, destruction of cellular membranes, and production of a variety of toxic chemicals, including prostaglandins, leucotrienes, and free radicals.

Iron Delocalization and Free-Radical Production. Following ischemia, sufficient free iron is released from ferritin to catalyze intracellular reactions that produce large amounts of free hydroxyl radicals. These free radicals are extremely reactive substances that attack proteins and lipid components of cells. This causes widespread lipid peroxidase chain reactions that alter molecular architecture. The accumulation of free iron and free radicals may create accelerating chain reactions that lead to widespread cell death. There is controversy, however, over whether these products have a significant role to play in tissue injury, or merely reflect the dissolution of cells that have died from other causes.

Uniform Theory of Ischemia-Induced Cellular Injury. The hypothesized calcium and iron disturbances just discussed have been combined to produce a uniform theory of ischemia-induced tissue injury. In this theory, the cellular calcium overloading triggers the release of free iron from intracellular storage sites. Both calcium and free iron catalyze reactions that form free radicals, resulting in the development of lipid peroxidation chain reactions, damage to cell membranes, and further release of free iron and calcium. The products of lipid peroxidation may cross the damaged cell membranes and enter the circulation. Secondary injury may thus be initiated in other organs that were not severely damaged by the initial ischemic insult. These observations support the concept that the post-resuscitation syndrome is a multi-organ syndrome in which other sick organs contribute to the pathophysiologic processes occurring in the brain, and the brain contributes to the pathophysiologic processes occurring in other organs.

The Major Determinants of Neurologic Outcome: Arrest Time and CPR Time. Success in both cardiac and brain resuscitation is inversely proportional to the duration of pulselessness without CPR (arrest time), and the time from the start of CPR until the restoration of a pulse (CPR time).

Arrest Time. Animal experiments have shown that the cerebral blood flow achieved with standard closed-chest CPR is affected by the duration of the arrest time that preceded the start of CPR. With cardiac arrest there is a continued loss of muscle tone in the heart, aorta, and arteries. Because of this loss of tone, there is a progressive decline in the ability of the chest compressions of CPR to produce blood flow. This is an important factor in both current theories about the mechanism of blood flow during CPR: the thoracic pump theory and the heart pump theory. Animal studies have demonstrated that after 2 minutes of "down" or arrest time, standard CPR produces 50% of normal cerebral blood flow; after 5 minutes of arrest time, this is reduced to 25–30% of normal flow; and after 10 minutes of arrest time, cerebral blood flow is zero with standard CPR.

CPR Time. As noted above, the effectiveness of CPR is markedly limited by the duration of the preceding arrest time. CPR must be started early, or its effectiveness is lost. Similarly, CPR effectiveness deteriorates markedly the longer it is continued. CPR does not sustain indefinitely the ability of the patient to be resuscitated. The longer the duration of CPR before a perfusing rhythm is restored, the worse the chances of survival. The purpose of closed-chest CPR is to provide some artificial circulation to the myocardium until electrical countershock can be administered to eliminate ventricular fibrillation. CPR only prolongs the process of dying—it buys time until the arrival of the defibrillator and the other elements of advanced cardiac care.

The "Low-Flow Versus No-Flow" Controversy. Standard closed-chest CPR is thought, at best, to generate only 20–30% of normal cardiac output. Nonetheless, there is overwhelming clinical evidence that despite these low flow levels, standard CPR has beneficial effects on both survival and neurologic recovery. Studies of prehospital cardiac arrest in particular have confirmed that early CPR, started by citizens who witnessed the arrest, contributes to improved survival.

Some laboratory data exist, however, that stand in opposition to much of the clinical data. There are animal studies that suggest that the low flow produced by standard CPR should not have a positive clinical benefit. According to these observations, the "trickle flow" produced by standard CPR may actually be a level of blood flow that is *more* damaging than no blood flow at all. In theory, anaerobic metabolism and lactate production cease after about 5 minutes of circulatory arrest. These processes, however, can continue if a trickle (less than 10–20% of normal) of brain blood flow is provided. The continued lactate production increases hydrogen ion concentration and worsens tissue acidosis. These progressive biochemical abnormalities may induce irreversible tissue damage. In contrast to these observations in animals, other studies have shown that residual flow during cerebral ischemia is better than no flow at all. The key seems to be whether or not hyperglycemia develops. High blood glucose levels contribute to the tissue lactic acid production. As long as blood glucose and tissue lactic acid concentrations do not rise unduly, a small degree of residual perfusion during ischemia seems to improve recovery.

Much of this so-called controversy stems from a mass of confusing and contradictory physiologic data. A variety of techniques have been used to attempt to accurately measure cerebral blood flow during closed-chest CPR. Different experimental models, different measurement techniques, and a variety of insult mechanisms and durations have yielded inconsistent estimates of cerebral blood flow. These estimates range from 1 to 60% of pre-arrest cerebral blood flow.

Although some biochemical and electrophysiologic parameters seem to be worsened during CPR-generated reperfusion, in the final clinical analysis the possibility of functional recovery is unquestionably increased with standard CPR.

THERAPEUTIC APPROACH TO BRAIN RESUSCITATION FOLLOWING CARDIAC ARREST

The therapeutic approach to brain resuscitation following cardiac arrest has two aspects: first, support of noncerebral organs; and second, brain-specific therapies. Although brain-specific therapies have attracted intensive research attention, at present, *no single brain-specific drug or therapeutic modality has been proved conclusively to be of benefit following global brain ischemia.* Even though several brain-specific therapies are discussed in this book, none are recommended at this time for routine clinical use. Only after reproducible animal studies have stimulated rigorous testing of promising brain resuscitation therapies in scientifically valid clinical trials should these therapies be recommended for widespread clinical use.

Nonetheless, the importance of providing general support of *noncerebral organs* during the post-ischemic period cannot be overemphasized and is the most effective brain-resuscitation therapy now available. Appreciation of this perspective has evolved through both laboratory and clinical investigations of brain-specific therapies. The general support of noncerebral organs is most effective when formalized into *standard brain-oriented intensive care protocols*.

Standard Brain-Oriented Intensive Care
(See Table 12–1)

1. Maintain Normotension Throughout Coma. After restoration of spontaneous circulation, arterial pressure should be rapidly normalized, using intravascular volume administration and vasopressors, as needed. There is normally an autoregulation of cerebral blood flow so that the flow remains constant despite blood pressures that can range from 50 to 150 mm Hg. During ischemia, however, this autoregulation is compromised, or even lost. Postischemic hypotension can cause severe compromise of cerebral blood flow and result in significant additional brain damage. Thus maintenance of adequate cerebral perfusion pressure in the normal to high-normal range (determined by the individual's pre-arrest blood pressure) is a mainstay of treatment.

Hypotension should be treated initially with plasma volume expansion, using either crystalloids (e.g., 10 ml/kg of lactate Ringer's solution) or colloids, as chosen by the clinician. Resistant hypotension should then be corrected by titrated IV infusion of dopamine. If this is not effective (i.e., >15 μg/kg/min is required), a norephinephrine or epinephrine IV infusion may be used, with further plasma volume expansion as indicated.

Severe arterial *hypertension* should also be quickly corrected by titrated IV infusion of a vasodilator (e.g., trimethaphan [Arfonad], nitroglycerin, or nitroprusside).

2. Correction of Acidosis: Arterial pH 7.3 to 7.5. Severe tissue lactic acidosis limits the possibility for cell survival after brain ischemia. Therapeutic measures aimed at ameliorating tissue acidosis are of significant benefit. A decrease in Pco_2 may compensate to some extent for metabolic acids that accumulate during ischemia. Respiratory compensation for a metabolic acid load, however, is limited. In addition, bicarbonate therapy, as currently recommended, may have detrimental cellular effects, since it is a CO_2 donor and can cause paradoxical CSF acidosis. Increased ventilation is mandatory to enable excretion of bicarbonate-generated CO_2. Correction of intracellular acidosis remains a therapeutic challenge.

3. Moderate Hyperventilation to Maintain Arterial Pco_2 Within Range of 25–35 mm Hg. Passive hyperventilation lowers arterial carbon dioxide tension, which in turn produces cerebral vasoconstriction. This vasoconstriction lowers the intracranial blood volume and effectively lowers intracranial pressure. This is a time-honored

Table 12–1. STANDARD BRAIN-ORIENTED INTENSIVE CARE

Every intensive care unit that treats patients resuscitated from cardiac arrest should adopt a strict brain-oriented resuscitation protocol. In several clinical trials, such a protocol has proved superior to nonprotocol "usual care." The features listed below have been part of these protocols. The independent effectiveness of each of these features is discussed in the text.

1. Maintain normotension throughout coma:
    a. Use IV vasopressor/vasodilator and fluids as needed
    b. Position head up 10–30°
2. Correct acidosis; maintain arterial pH of 7.3 to 7.5:
    a. Use ventilation and bicarbonate as needed
3. Moderate hyperventilation:
    a. Maintain arterial P_{CO_2} of 25–35 mm Hg during controlled ventilation
    b. Maintain arterial P_{CO_2} of 20–40 mm Hg during spontaneous breathing
4. Maintain arterial P_{O_2} greater than 100 mm Hg, while using the lowest possible FIO_2 and PEEP:
    a. FIO_2 90–100% at first
    b. After 1–6 hours, use FIO_2 50%
5. Immobilize and sedate the patient as needed:
    a. Use softening (not fully paralyzing) doses of relaxant (e.g., pancuronium IV) if necessary during controlled ventilation
6. Treat and prevent seizures:
    a. Thiopental or pentobarbital, 5 mg/kg/hr (aim for plasma level of 2–4 mg/dl); total: 30 mg/kg
                                    OR
    b. Phenytoin (10–15 mg/kg IV, loading dose; 7 mg/kg/24 h maintenance)
                                    OR
    c. Diazepam, 5 mg/70 kg IV, titrated as needed
7. Normalize the hematocrit and the blood chemistries:
    a. Hematocrit: 30–35% at least
    b. Serum osmolality: 280–330 mOsm/L
    c. Glucose: 100–300 mg/dl
8. Consider corticosteroids based upon local standard of care:
    a. Methylprednisolone, 1 mg/kg IV, followed by 0.5 mg/kg/6 h IV
                                    OR
    Dexamethasone, 0.2 mg/kg IV, followed by 0.1 mg/kg/6 h IV
    b. Stop or taper corticosteroids at 48–72 hours
9. Maintain normothermia; avoid hyperthermia
10. Initiate osmotherapy for *monitored* increases in intracranial pressure or for secondary neurologic deterioration
    a. Monitor intracranial pressure only if safe technique established. This is optional after CPR; recommended after cerebral trauma
    b. Mannitol, 0.5 g/kg IV, can be given empirically, without ICP monitoring, immediately following restoration of spontaneous circulation after cardiac arrest, and upon noting signs of neurologic deterioration
11. Place patient in a 10–30° upright position
12. Start nutritional support by 48 hours
13. Institute regular CNS evaluations

and effective method of treating head-injured patients with swollen brains from vasogenic edema. Most patients, however, do not develop a continued elevation of intracranial pressure after cardiac arrest, despite the cytotoxic cellular edema that is known to occur. Therefore, hyperventilation would not be expected to benefit most post–cardiac arrest patients by this mechanism.

Though hyperventilation is partially effective in correction of post-ischemic tissue acidosis, this effect begins to gradually decline after about 4 hours. In addition, the "reverse steal" phenomenon, in which hyperventilation causes vasoconstriction of normal blood vessels with a shunting of blood to more severely affected areas, is currently considered a doubtful possibility. Other than the exceptions of patients with vasogenic edema and intracranial hypertension from late secondary neurologic deterioration, passive hyperventilation is of unproved value for the comatose cardiac arrest survivor. Nonetheless, the use of hyperventilation to ensure that the PCO_2 remains in the range of 25–35 mm Hg seems clinically reasonable.

4. Maintain Oxygenation: Arterial Po_2 >100 mm Hg with lowest possible FIO_2 and PEEP. Adequate tissue oxygenation preserves cellular function and allows post-ischemic reparative processes to take place. Transient pulmonary problems could cause deterioration in the oxygenation of already compromised tissues. Arterial Po_2 levels should be maintained using the lowest FIO_2 possible, with carefully titrated levels of PEEP. Adjust the ventilator tidal volume, frequency, and flow rate to achieve optimal lung compliance, arterial Po_2, arterial Pco_2, and alveolar-arterial oxygen gradient. Avoid causing circulatory depression. Recent concerns that high arterial oxygen levels generate injurious free radicals are speculative and should not affect current clinical practice.

5. Immobilize and Sedate as Necessary. External stimuli increase cerebral metabolism at a time when the oxygen demand/supply ratio is already precariously balanced. Administration of *titrated doses* of sedative/anesthetic drugs (e.g., diazepam, 2–5 mg IV, or phenobarbital, 2–5 mg/kg, repeated as needed) and "softening" doses of muscle relaxants (e.g., pancuronium, 0.05 mg/kg, repeated as needed) will protect the patient from afferent sensory impulses, prevent oxygen demand/supply imbalance, and improve the chances for neuronal recovery.

6. Treat and Prevent Seizures. There is controversy about the prophylactic (i.e., before a seizure occurs) use of anticonvulsant drugs. Once seizures occur, however, they should be quickly and effectively treated. Seizure activity can increase brain metabolism by 300 to 400%. This extreme increase in metabolic demand may tip the oxygen demand/supply balance unfavorably, with harmful neurologic consequences. Commonly used drugs include barbiturates, phenytoin, and diazepam. Phenytoin has been reported also to improve neurologic recovery, through a membrane stabilization mechanism rather than through its anticonvulsant effect. Further study is needed, however, before its use can be recommended for this effect alone.

Seizure activity (clinical or on EEG) should be controlled immediately when it occurs, using one of the following:

a. Intravenous diazepam in 5-mg increments, for immediate control of seizures.

b. Intravenous phenytoin loading, under continuous ECG monitoring, for all patients with seizures. Administration of phenytoin should not be faster than 50 mg/min, to a total dose of 15 mg/kg. After loading, administer maintenance doses of 200 mg phenytoin/70 kg/12 h. If monitoring of phenytoin plasma levels is possible, note that a level of 10–20 μg/ml is therapeutic. Recurrence of seizure activity during phenytoin therapy should be controlled with additional diazepam as in (a).

c. If cardiovascular complications occur during phenytoin loading or if the diazepam-phenytoin sequence fails to control seizures, intravenous phenobarbital should be used. The loading dose is 100–200 mg IV every 15 min, to a total of 15 mg/kg.

7. Normalization of Hematocrit and Blood Chemistries. The oxygen-carrying capacity of the blood should be maintained by an adequate hematocrit. The difficulty of balancing improvement of blood viscosity by hemodilution against the associated compromise of the oxygen-carrying capacity of the blood has not been resolved. High pre-ischemic blood glucose levels have been demonstrated to exacerbate post-reperfusion brain damage. Nevertheless, adequate nutritional support and at least normal post-resuscitation blood glucose levels should be maintained to supply needed metabolic substrates for tissue repair. Serum electrolytes, osmolality, pH, and other blood chemistries should be kept within normal ranges.

8. Corticosteroids. The value of corticosteroids administered after cardiac arrest is unproved. Despite lack of documented efficacy, there are a number of proposed effects of steroids (e.g., membrane stabilization, reactivation of $Na+/K+$ membrane pump) that contribute some rationale to their continued widespread clinical use.

However, there are also possible risks associated with even short-term use of steroids (48–72 hours), especially for the patient with an acute MI. We consider steroids at present to be an optional therapeutic intervention. If used, a reasonable regimen would be dexamethasone, 0.2 mg/kg IV, as soon as possible, followed by 0.1 mg/kg every 6 hours.

9. Maintain Normothermia. Elevation of temperature above normal can cause significant imbalance between oxygen supply and demand by increasing brain metabolism at a time when cerebral blood flow is compromised. It should be aggressively treated in the post-ischemic period.

In contrast, hypothermia is the most effective method known for suppression of cerebral metabolic activity. Hypothermia, however, has significant detrimental effects, such as increased blood viscosity, decreased cardiac output, and increased susceptibility to infection. Additionally, hypothermia is a difficult therapeutic modality to implement clinically. It is not recommended for routine clinical use after cardiac arrest.

10. Osmotherapy. Not recommended for routine clinical use after cardiac arrest. However, if intracranial pressure is *monitored* and elevation of the intracranial pressure is documented, titrated administration of mannitol, 0.25–0.5 gm/kg, may be useful. Serum osmolality should be monitored frequently. The development of secondary neurologic deterioration may also be an indication for osmotherapy.

Intracranial pressure would be monitored where feasible and when an ICP rise is clinically suspected. In cases of secondary CNS deterioration, which can be seen at 24–72 hours post arrest, ICP (if monitored) should be kept below 15 mm Hg with the following sequential measures: (1) hyperventilation to $Paco_2$ of 20–25 mm Hg; (2) venting of CSF; (3) osmotherapy with mannitol; (4) thiopental or pentobarbital in titrated IV anesthetic doses. A loop diuretic may be added as an adjunctive treatment (major effect is to decrease CSF production—a delayed effect on ICP).

11. Patient Position. Patient positioning is directed toward reducing cerebral venous pressure. The head and upper body should be elevated 10–30 degrees to promote venous drainage, particularly during PEEP therapy. Torsion or compression of the neck veins should be avoided by not rotating or flexing the head, and by elimination of compressive dressings. Frequent turning of the patient from side to side will help prevent atelectasis.

12. Nutritional Support. Adequate nutritional support through oral intake, nasogastric tube feedings, or parenteral hyperalimentation should begin within 48 hours. This supplies the metabolic substrates that are necessary for post-ischemic tissue repair.

13. Fluid Balance. Fluid balance should be controlled as clinically indicated. Avoid use of pure dextrose-in-water and overhydration, which may exacerbate cerebral edema.

14. Cardiovascular Monitoring. This should include monitoring of both arterial pressure (by cuff or preferably with an intra-arterial catheter) and central venous pressure, during flow and ECG. Monitoring of pulmonary artery/wedge pressures, cardiac output, and systemic vascular resistance (SVR) should be instituted as clinically indicated.

15. CNS Evaluation. Continuous careful bedside monitoring of neurologic function, using simple but relevant clinical tools such as the Glasgow and Glasgow-Pittsburgh Coma scores (Table 12–2),

Table 12–2. GLASGOW-PITTSBURGH COMA SCORE

Glasgow Coma Score

NOTE: If patient is under the influence of anesthetics, sedatives, or neuromuscular blockers, give best estimate of each item.
Write number in box to indicate status at time of exam

(A) EYE OPENING ☐
Spontaneous	= 4
To speech	= 3
To pain	= 2
None	= 1

(B) BEST MOTOR RESPONSE ☐
(extremities or best side)
Obeys	= 6
Localizes	= 5
Withdraws	= 4
Abnormal flexion	= 3
Extends	= 2
None	= 1

(C) BEST VERBAL RESPONSE ☐
(if patient intubated, give best estimate)
Oriented	= 5
Confused conversation	= 4
Inappropriate words	= 3
Incomprehensible sounds	= 2
None	= 1

Pittsburgh Brain Stem Score

Check appropriate box for each item.

	(1) YES	(2) NO
Lash and/or corneal reflex present (either side)	☐	☐
Doll's eye and/or ice water calories present (either side)	☐	☐
Right pupil reacts to light	☐	☐
Left pupil reacts to light	☐	☐
Gag and/or cough reflex present	☐	☐

The primary purpose of this scoring system is to identify a hierarchical *level* of function from brain stem to cerebrum, not to indicate laterality of disease.

helps to monitor changes in patient condition and improve therapeutic decision-making. Use *EEG monitoring* (optional) by standard technique or cerebral function monitor (CFM) as clinically indicated.

Brain-Specific Therapies

The most effective therapeutic regimen currently available—meticulous adherence to a carefully designed brain-oriented therapeutic protocol—has already been discussed. The brain-specific therapies discussed below are largely experimental approaches.

None are currently recommended for routine clinical use in patients following cardiac arrest.

1. Barbiturates. Barbiturates have appeared promising because of their ability to reduce cerebral metabolism, edema formation, intracranial pressure, seizure activity, and the damage induced by focal and incomplete ischemia. Randomized clinical trials of high-dose (up to 30 mg/kg) barbiturates were conducted with comatose cardiac survivors in the late 1970s and early 1980s. These studies confirmed the value of *standard, brain-oriented intensive care,* but demonstrated no significant improvement in neurologic outcomes for the patients who received barbiturates. This high-dose barbiturate loading cannot, therefore, be recommended for routine clinical use after cardiac arrest. Nevertheless, the studies demonstrated that when the specific and proved therapeutic effects of barbiturates are desired, such as sedation, anticonvulsant action, or intracranial pressure reduction, the drugs can, in skilled hands, be safely administered to this group of patients.

2. Calcium-Entry Blocking Drugs. In the wake of expanding clinical popularity as well as the unfolding calcium-related pathophysiology of brain ischemia, investigators have begun to examine the potential usefulness of calcium-entry blocking agents after circulatory arrest. In animals pretreated with calcium channel blockers prior to prolonged ischemic brain insults, a preservation of cellular architecture and an almost complete protection against cellular calcium influx has been demonstrated. Post-insult administration of these agents after global brain ischemia has demonstrated a significant beneficial effect in a variety of animal models, using differing drugs and dosages. Under NIH support, 25 hospitals in 12 countries are now testing the efficacy of lidoflazine, an investigational calcium entry blocker, to improve neurologic recovery in comatose cardiac arrest survivors. Final results are expected in 1987.

3. Prostaglandin Inhibitors and Thromboxane Antagonists. After ischemia, destruction of cell membranes releases free fatty acids, which are metabolized to prostaglandins, thromboxanes, and other cytotoxic substances. Though studies in stroke patients with indomethacin (a prostaglandin synthesis inhibitor) and prostacyclin (a thromboxane antagonist) have been promising, no clinical experience exists with the use of these drugs after cardiac arrest.

4. Free Radical Scavengers. Free radicals, substances with unpaired electrons in outer orbital rings, are highly reactive substances generated during ischemia-induced degradation of lipids. Though their significance in ischemic cell death is unclear, free radical scavengers such as superoxide dismutase, ascorbic acid, vitamin E, and DMSO have recently received a great deal of clinical interest. No definitive studies are yet available.

5. Free Iron Chelators. The accumulation of intracellular free iron released during prolonged ischemia is thought to stimulate several processes that can destroy cell membranes. Free iron chelators, such as desferoxamine, can bind iron and keep it chemically inert, thus inhibiting the intracellular destructive processes of lipid peroxidation and free radical formation. Investigations are in preliminary stages, and the clinical application of early findings is uncertain.

6. Miscellaneous Therapies. A number of experimental brain resuscitation therapies, of varying potential promise, still await definitive investigation. These include:

Naloxone: Reported in some studies to significantly improve ischemic neurologic deficits in animals and man. Other studies have failed to demonstrate benefit.

Dimethyl Sulfoxide: An industrial organic solvent that scavenges free radicals, reduces platelet aggregation, and stabilizes lysosomal membranes. A brain-protective effect has not been established.

Cardiopulmonary Bypass: A beneficial effect after prolonged cardiac arrest has been demonstrated in animal experimental work. Use of such an approach on an emergency basis may allow restoration of spontaneous circulation in patients refractory to standard CPR and ACLS, with improved reperfusion of the brain and amelioration of post-ischemic brain damage. Administration of potentially brain-benefiting pharmacologic interventions with cardiovascular depressent side effects would be easily implemented with this control of circulation.

CONCLUSION

The search continues for effective clinical interventions to limit neurologic damage after severe global brain ischemia. Ongoing systematic investigations should lead to the development of one or, more likely, a series of brain-benefiting therapies. These therapies will ultimately be implemented in a multifaceted therapeutic protocol to restore "healthy minds in healthy bodies."

REFERENCES

1. Levy DE, Bates D, Caronna JJ, et al: Prognosis in nontraumatic coma. Ann Intern Med *94*:293, 1981.
2. Graham DI: The pathology of brain ischemia and possibilities for therapeutic intervention. Br J Anaesth *57*:3, 1985.
3. White BC, Winegar CP, Henderson O, et al: Prolonged "no-reflow" in the dog's cerebral cortex after cardiac arrest. Ann Emerg Med *12*:414, 1983.
4. McCord JM: Oxygen derived free radicals in post-ischemic tissue injury. N Engl J Med *312*:159, 1985.

5. Safar P: Recent advances in cardiopulmonary-cerebral resuscitation. Ann Emerg Med *13*(Part 2):856, 1984.
6. Abramson NS, Safar P, Detre KM, et al: Neurologic recovery after cardiac arrest: effect of duration of ischemia. Crit Care Med *13*:361A, 1985.
7. Gisvold SE, Steen PA: Drug therapy in brain ischemia. Br J Anaesth *57*:96, 1985.
8. Abramson NS, Safar P, Detre KM, et al: Randomized clinical study of cardio-pulmonary-cerebral resuscitation: thiopental loading in comatose cardiac arrest survivors. N Engl J Med *314*:397, 1986.
9. Kelsey SF, Abramson NS, Detre KM, et al: Randomized clinical study of cardiopulmonary-cerebral resuscitation: design, methods and patient characteristics. Am J Emerg Med *4*:72, 1986.
10. Safar P: On the evolution of brain resuscitation. Crit Care Med *6*:199, 1978.
11. Levy DR, Caronna JJ, Singer BH, et al: Predicting outcome for hypoxic-ischemia coma. JAMA *253*:1420, 1985.
12. Fishman RA: Steroids in the treatment of brain edema. N Engl J Med *306*:359, 1982.
13. Mullie A, Abramson NS, Safar P, et al: Clinical studies of thiopental loading after cardiac arrest (Abstract). Crit Care Med *9*:194, 1981.

13

PEDIATRIC CARDIAC ARREST

Primary cardiac arrest in infants and small children without congenital or acquired heart disease is a relatively uncommon event. The vast majority of pediatric arrests are primary respiratory arrests due to airway obstruction and hypoxia. Reversal of a respiratory arrest through rapid establishment of a patent airway is generally associated with a good prognosis, with an overall mortality rate of approximately 25%.

Secondary cardiac arrests in children are usually the result of prolonged respiratory arrest and are associated with severe neurologic sequelae and poor prognoses, with an overall mortality rate of approximately 90%. A number of minutes of apnea (mean of 17 minutes) must transpire before asystole occurs in a child.

Terminal dysrhythmias in infants and small children tend to be brady-dysrhythmias secondary to hypoxia, progressing to asystole if the hypoxia is not reversed. The small heart muscle cannot propagate and maintain ventricular fibrillation. As the age of the child increases, the incidence of ventricular dysrhythmias associated with cardiac arrest increases. A defibrillator is not considered a mandatory piece of equipment on many infant care units or transport vehicles, owing to the low incidence of ventricular dys-rhythmias. On the other hand, defibrillators are usually considered routine on pediatric care units.

CAUSES OF RESPIRATORY ARREST IN CHILDREN

Acute Airway Obstruction

The most common life-threatening causes of airway obstruction in the small child are epiglottitis and foreign body aspiration. Other conditions that may cause acute airway obstruction are choanal atresia, congenital webs, and Pierre Robin syndrome. Any condition that can cause edema, narrowing, or occlusion of the airway, such as tumors or asthma, may also place the child at risk for airway obstruction and possible respiratory arrest.

Foreign Body Aspiration

The child with foreign body aspiration may present acutely with complete airway obstruction and require removal of the object or tracheostomy to bypass the object. Partial airway obstruction may

163

present hours or days later, accompanied by pneumonia. Clearly, the child with complete airway obstruction is most at risk for cardiopulmonary arrest if the obstruction is not relieved rapidly. Since most cases of complete airway obstruction occur out of the hospital, prognosis will depend heavily on the actions of the initial care givers. Treatment would include head positioning, finger sweep, back blows, and chest thrusts as described in the American Heart Association recommendations.

Epiglottitis

Children with suspected epiglottitis should receive supplemental cool-mist oxygen and rapid radiologic evaluation. Direct visualization of the epiglottis should be carried out only in a controlled operating room setting, preferably with both an anesthesiologist and an ENT physician in attendance, should endotracheal intubation be necessary. Tracheostomy is now rarely performed if prompt recognition is accompanied with rapid and skilled intubation in a controlled hospital setting.

If personnel skilled in the management of acute airway obstruction in the child are not readily available, attempts should be made to keep the child as calm and comfortable as possible until help arrives. The child should be allowed to assume the position he or she desires—usually upright and near or in a parent's arms. Painful procedures should be delayed, to prevent crying and further deterioration of the airway.

Central Nervous System Depression

Electrical shock, hypoxia and/or hypercapnia, infections, and trauma are examples of conditions that can cause increased intracranial pressure and cerebral edema, which may lead to respiratory arrest in children. *Trauma* (typically from head injury, near drowning, and/or strangulation) and *infections* (usually meningitis, encephalitis, or Reye's syndrome*) are most often responsible for respiratory arrest in small children in this category.

Signs and symptoms of increased intracranial pressure in the toddler up to age 18 months may be subtle and thus difficult to identify in light of significant cerebral edema. This is because the anterior fontanel does not close until age 16–18 months and acts as an intrinsic "pop-off" mechanism, allowing the brain to swell proportionately more than an adult's, with fewer overt symptoms and sequelae.

---

*There has been a steady decline in the number of reported cases of Reye's syndrome since 1985; this is thought to be due to the increased caution associated with aspirin administration.

Mechanical Impairment of Ventilation

Infections (e.g., botulism, Guillain-Barré syndrome, diphtheria, and polio), paralyzing drugs, myasthenia gravis, phrenic nerve palsy, and spinal cord trauma can all result in neuromuscular paralysis and subsequent respiratory arrest due to mechanical impairment of ventilation.

Restriction of Ventilation

In the small child, trauma to the chest wall and iatrogenic insults to the airway may occur. Chest wall trauma is usually secondary to child abuse or motor vehicle accidents.

Iatrogenic insults may include right mainstem bronchus intubation and esophageal intubation. The relatively short length of the child's airway in contrast to the relatively long length of uncut endotracheal tubes increases the risk of right mainstem intubation. A thin chest wall and increased sound transmission commonly mislead the intubator to believe the trachea has been intubated when in fact an esophageal intubation has taken place.

Gastric distention can also severely restrict ventilation and is often overlooked until the child becomes symptomatic. Symptoms include vomiting and/or aspiration, abdominal perforation, and hypoxia and/or hypercarbia.

Endotracheal tube obstruction due to inadequate maintenance can also cause complete restriction of ventilation. Because of the small internal diameters of pediatric endotracheal tubes, a minimal decrease in the airway diameter from secretions can cause disproportionate airway resistance and compromise.

Parenchymal Disease

Pulmonary edema, atelectasis, and surfactant failure (respiratory distress syndromes and near drowning) contribute most often to respiratory compromise and arrest in the pediatric population. Infants and small children also have fewer collateral ventilatory pathways and may suffer significant distress from seemingly small amounts of atelectasis.

CAUSES OF CARDIAC ARREST IN CHILDREN

Vagal Stimulation

One of the most common causes of brady-dysrhythmias and subsequent inadequate cardiac output in children is vagal stimulation. It is frequently associated with endotracheal intubation/extubation, gastric tube insertion, or suctioning of the airway.

Shock

Hypovolemic shock, usually secondary to dehydrative states or hemorrhage, is the most common cause of shock in the small child. Early recognition of shock states in children is often extremely difficult because of intact compensatory mechanisms and a relative lack of overt symptoms initially. For example, a child can lose 20% of circulating blood volume and experience only a slight tachycardia. Hypotension is a late symptom in a child and must be treated aggressively when present.

Septic (vasogenic) shock is the second most common type, followed by *cardiogenic shock*. Signs and symptoms may be extremely subtle initially. By the time hypotension is present, the child appears critically ill and requires massive fluid resuscitation and vasopressor support.

Congenital Heart Disease

Cardiac failure may result from complications associated with transposition of the great vessels and Stokes-Adams disease secondary to congenital AV block. Iatrogenic heart block following surgical repair of a congenital heart defect can also predispose children to cardiac arrest. There are an increasing number of children who suffer sudden cardiac death, sometimes years after surgical repair of their heart defect. These cases appear to be related to residual and/or increasing left ventricular outflow tract obstruction, pulmonary valvular disease, and heart block.

Severe congestive heart failure may result from unrepaired coarctation of the aorta, critical aortic stenosis, pulmonary stenosis, patent ductus arteriosus, and large ventricular septal defects. Any time an infant or child presents with severe CHF, the above conditions should be considered as a possible etiology.

Acquired Heart Disease

Infections such as myocarditis, endocarditis, rheumatic heart disease, and Kawasaki disease may contribute to cardiac compromise. Aneurysm formation and myocardial infarction secondary to Kawasaki disease are responsible for the 1.5–2% mortality rate associated with the disease.

Miscellaneous Causes

Hypothermia, hypoglycemia, diabetic ketoacidosis, and massive air embolism are other possible causes of cardiac arrest in small children.

BASIC LIFE SUPPORT

The single most important factor affecting prognosis in pediatric arrest states is early recognition of "pre-arrest" states. This is not always easy, because of the excellent compensatory mechanisms, subtlety of symptoms, and lack of cognitive communication skills seen in small children. Portions of the history and physical exam, combined with one's "gut feelings" regarding the diagnosis, may help in identifying pre-arrest states.

Airway

Establishing an effective airway may be all that is necessary to prevent respiratory arrest. The child's head should be positioned in a neutral or "sniffing" position, with only slight elevation under the shoulders or occiput. Hyperextension can compromise or collapse the young child's cartilaginous trachea and actually obstruct the airway.

The proportionally larger tongues in children may require jaw-thrust maneuver to lift the tongue up and out of the airway if the "sniffing" position is not effective. Because aspiration is a common cause of airway obstruction, the oral cavity should be inspected for foreign bodies, formula, secretions, etc., and suctioned if necessary. In the event that suctioning equipment is not readily available, a finger sweep through the posterior oropharynx should be performed if the obstruction can be visualized. The head should be positioned to the side if the child is vomiting, to decrease the chance of aspiration.

There are some situations in which endotracheal intubation is necessary for airway protection when the airway is compromised secondary to swelling or trauma.

Breathing

Ventilation should be assisted whenever *effective* breathing ceases. This includes cases in which the patient is still breathing but exhibits cyanosis, wheezing, stridor, grunting, flaring, retracting, signs of acidosis, and so on. In the past, there has been an unfortunate tendency to withhold rescue breathing until there is no respiration. However, today it is recognized that the importance of supportive measures and recognition of "pre-arrest" states cannot be stressed enough. Early intervention through supportive therapy (e.g., head/body position, cool-mist oxygen, and other measures) may be all that is required to prevent a complete respiratory arrest.

Circulation

In the majority of pediatric arrests, the establishment of an adequate airway and effective ventilation is all that is required. Because hypoxia and concomitant hypoxemia are often responsible for bradycardia and hypotension in children, correction of hypoxia may prevent cardiac arrest.

Circulation should be supported when it is no longer adequate—not after it ceases. Circulation is inadequate if associated with an abnormal level of consciousness, tachycardia, cool, mottled extremities, decreased urine output, hypotension, weak or absent pulses, and/or acidosis. In addition, a "normal" heart rate does not always mean that there is adequate circulation. Pulse validation and assessment of the above-mentioned indicators of cardiac output should all be considered when assessing the child with compromised circulation.

If the heart rate is not supporting adequate cardiac output or there is absent cardiac output, cardiac compressions should be instituted. There is often a hesitancy to begin external compressions when a heart rate is present. The criteria for support must not be based upon whether a heart rate is present or not but rather on whether there is adequate cardiac output.

ADVANCED LIFE SUPPORT

Once the basics of CPR are started, attention can be turned toward advanced treatment with artificial airways, medications, and defibrillation.

Endotracheal Intubation

1. Premedication with atropine is commonly used to prevent bradycardia due to vagal response and/or to combat the side effects of paralytic agents such as Anectine. Often, complete paralysis is indicated in the infant or child who is likely to fight the procedure. However, paralytic agents should be administered only when respiration can be supported via bag/mask in the event the intubation attempt is unsuccessful.

2. Tube sizes should be chosen appropriate to weight (see Table 13–1 for tube sizes). Children under 8 years of age do not require cuffed endotracheal tubes, owing to the natural narrowing of the trachea at the cricoid ring. Older children have an airway similar to adults in that the vocal cords are the narrowest point, thus requiring cuffed tubes.

3. Endotracheal tube placement should be confirmed via chest x-ray as well as documentation of bilateral breath sounds, mist in the ET tube, and chest motion with manual ventilation.

4. Nasal endotracheal tubes are easier to stabilize in small children, as they are not subjected to tube biting or copious oral secretion (see Figs. 13–1 and 13–2 for oral and nasal ET tube taping techniques). Maintenance of tube patency must be addressed, owing to the small ET tube diameters and increased chance of occlusion. Warm, humidified oxygen should be administered via ventilator or aerosol tubing with a T-piece. Suctioning should be performed every 2–3 hours to ensure tube patency.

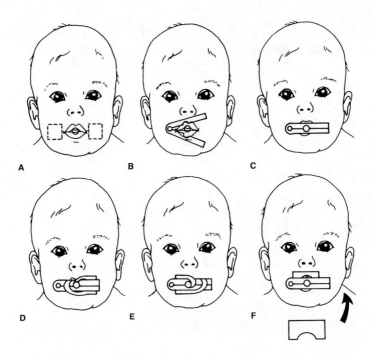

1. Apply benzoin or Tegaderm to face (A). (Do not use both together, as removal is difficult.)

2. Umbi clamp the endotracheal tube (B, C) with the appropriately sized drill hole (hole should be drilled the size of the external diameter of desired tube size).

3. Cut piece of 1″ tape into a 5″ segment, make into a U shape:

(a)	
(b)	

   (a) Wrap top half of tape around tube, circling tube from top side (D).
   (b) Wrap bottom half of tape around umbi clamp from bottom side (D).

4. Repeat #3 from opposite side (E).

5. Optional: Cut an upside-down mustache piece of tape and place it under the umbi clamp to secure taping (F).

Figure 13–1. Taping orotracheal tubes using umbilical clamp securement (used for ET tube sizes 3.0–4.5).

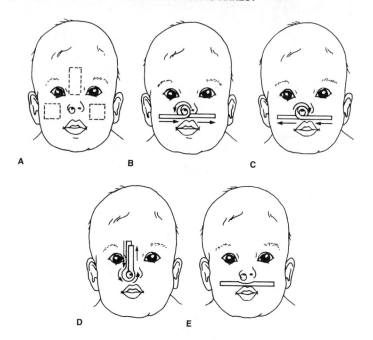

1. Apply benzoin or Tegaderm to face (A). (Do not use both together, as removal is difficult.)

2. Cut 3 pieces of ½″ tape (approximately 6–8″ long). It is always better to have a long piece of tape than to be caught "short" in the middle of taping the ET tube!

3. Place the first piece of tape on the right cheek bone and draw across the bottom of the tube, circling (2 complete revolutions) counterclockwise (B). Take excess tape and secure to left cheekbone.

4. Repeat #3, starting on left cheekbone, and reverse procedure, circling clockwise with second piece of tape (C).

5. Take third piece of tape from forehead down bridge of nose. Wrap tape around tube, bringing excess tape back up over bridge of nose (D).

6. Optional: Cut upside-down mustache piece of tape and place across upper lip to secure taping (E).

Figure 13–2. Taping nasotracheal tubes.

5. Gastric tubes must be considered adjunctive airway equipment when intubation or prolonged mask ventilation is required (see Table 13–1 for tube sizes). Because of the small abdominal capacity, a minimal amount of air can significantly distend the abdomen and cause elevation of the diaphragm, preventing effective ventilation.

Breathing

1. There have been many suggested rates and volumes recommended for assisted ventilation in small children over the years. In general, a rate of 15–40 ventilations per minute and volumes of 10 cc/kg can be used for children. NOTE: These are only guideline numbers and should be adjusted according to patient response.

2. 100% FIO_2 should always be delivered in an arrest situation, to promote oxygenation.

Circulation

1. Hand placement should always be on the lower third of the sternum, regardless of age. In the past, it was thought that hand placement should be on the middle third of the sternum for infants, but this has now been shown to be less effective, and the lower third is recommended for infants as well.

2. There have been many recommended rates for cardiac compressions in children over the past few decades. A rate of 100–140 per minute and compression depths adequate to generate femoral pulses should be used. NOTE: These are only guideline numbers and should be adjusted according to patient response. (Adequate patient response is indicated by a palpable pulse and blood pressure generation.)

3. Palpation of femoral or radial pulses is a rapid and effective way of assessing cardiac output during CPR.

Defibrillation/Cardioversion

1. As previously noted, defibrillation is rarely required during resuscitation of infants and children, owing to the infrequency of ventricular dysrhythmias (exceptions being in medical centers where heart surgery is performed). In the event of prolonged or supraventricular tachycardia or atrial fibrillation/flutter that has not responded to medical management and with evidence of decreased cardiac output, synchronized electrical cardioversion is indicated.

    a. For ventricular fibrillation or ventricular tachycardia without pulses, use *countershock*. Begin at 1 joule/kg; double dosage if ineffective.

    b. For ventricular tachycardia with pulses, supraventricular tachycardia, or atrial fibrillation/flutter, use *cardioversion*. Begin with 0.5 joule/kg and increase by doubling the dose.

2. Hypoxia/acidosis may prevent effective defibrillation.

3. Anterior-posterior paddle placement may be required for the child with an enlarged myocardium.

4. Care must be taken to avoid bony areas of the chest.

5. Paddle size should be the largest that will allow *complete* contact with the chest.

Table 13–1. TUBE SIZES AND IV SITES IN INFANTS AND CHILDREN

Age	Average Weight (kg)	ET Tube Size	Suction Catheter (Fr)	NG Tube Size (Fr)	Peripheral IV Size (ga)	Peripheral IV Site	Central IV Size	Central IV Site
1 mo	5	3.5	6	10	24, 22	Scalp, hand/arm, foot	*Ages 1 mo–2 yr:* 21 ga needle 3.0 Fr catheter 0.018 guide wire	Internal jugular or femoral vein used for all age groups listed
6 mo	7	3.5	6	10	24, 22, 20	Scalp, hand/arm, foot		
1 yr	10	4.0	8	12	22, 20	Hand, arm, foot		
2 yr	12	4.5	8	12	22, 20	Hand, arm, foot		
3 yr	14	4.5	8	12	22, 20	Hand, arm, foot	*Ages 3–13 yr:* 20 ga needle 4.0 Fr catheter 0.021 guide wire	
4 yr	16	5	10	12	22, 20	Hand, arm, foot		
5 yr	18	5	10	12	22, 20	Hand, arm, foot		
6 yr	20	5.5	10	12, 14	22, 20, 18	Hand, arm, foot		
7 yr	22	6	10	12, 14	22, 20, 18	Hand, arm, foot		
8 yr	24	6 cuff	10	12, 14	22, 20, 18	Hand, arm		
9 yr	26	6 cuff	10	12, 14	20, 18	Hand, arm		
10 yr	30	6.5 cuff	10	14	18	Hand, arm		
13 yr	40	7 cuff	14	16	18	Hand, arm		

6. Because of the small chest size of children, bridging may occur with the use of conductive gels. For this reason, pregelled pads are recommended, with care taken to let any excess hang over the sides of the chest.

Adjunctive Medications for Endotracheal Intubation

Anectine (Succinylcholine Chloride)
  Dosage: 1–2 mg/kg IV.
  Duration: 10–15 minutes.
  Contraindications: Patients with severe trauma (crush injuries), severe burns, eye injuries, myotonia, active myositis, cord transections, uncontrolled renal failure.
  Precautions: Precede with atropine (0.02 mg/kg IV), as Anectine can cause bradycardia in infants and children.
  NOTE: Administering Anectine to the patient with any of the listed contraindications can cause a sudden release of potassium to the point of producing a hyperkalemic cardiac arrest.

Pavulon (Pancuronium Chloride)
  Dosage: 0.1 mg/kg IV.
  Duration: 30–60 minutes.
  Precautions: Must be prepared and able to assist ventilation for duration of drug effect.

Valium (Diazepam)
  Dosage: 0.1 mg/kg IV.
  Duration: 30–60 minutes; onset occurs within 5 minutes if given IV.
  Precautions: Large doses may cause apnea.

INTRAVENOUS ACCESS IN THE PEDIATRIC PATIENT

It is important to establish a route by which medications can be delivered but also important not to waste precious time while doing so. Most pediatric arrests are respiratory arrests; thus, supporting the airway first may give personnel time to establish intravenous access. Some resuscitative medications can be administered via the endotracheal tube if necessary.

Peripheral Access

Sites

1. **1–6 Months.** Infants have many superficial veins located in the scalp that are relatively easy to cannulate. During an arrest

situation, however, these sites are prone to catheter dislodgment and infiltration. The back of the hand, antecubital veins, and saphenous veins are the most desirable sites.

2. 6 Months–2 Years. Often this age group can be the most difficult in which to establish intravenous access, owing to the presence of "baby fat," which obscures vein visibility. The saphenous vein, antecubital vein, and the back of the hand are the optimum sites. A site that is often forgotten is the anterior aspect of the forearm, which is usually quite free of "baby fat," so that veins are easily seen. It is also easy to restrain and secure this area.

3. 2–8 Years. The sites are the same as for an adult. Lower extremity sites are still utilized. The external jugular vein is relatively accessible at this age.

4. 8 Years and Older. The sites are the same as for an adult. Lower extremity sites are usually avoided because of the risk of phlebitis.

Types and Sizes of Catheters

1. Butterfly Needles. Sizes range from 25- to 19-gauge. Butterfly needles are useful for short-term administration of fluids and blood drawing. They are not recommended for long-term use, as they tend to infiltrate easily and to become dislodged unless anchored securely. Butterfly needles should not be used during cardiac arrest, as other types of needles provide better routes for fluids and medications. If necessary to employ them in this setting, however, it should be for short-term use only; another vein needs to be cannulated with a more stable plastic catheter as soon as possible.

2. Plastic Over-the-Needle Catheters. Sizes range from 24- to 12-gauge. These catheters are most useful for peripheral access. It is often assumed that small patients need small catheters. However, it is possible to place an 18-gauge catheter in a 5 year old. Always use the largest bore catheter that the vein will accept. These catheters are secured easily and will last about 3 days, depending upon the type of fluid or medications infused.

Central Vein Access (See Fig. 13–3)

Sites

1. 1–6 Months. It is difficult to obtain central venous access in infants, owing to the small size of the patient and the relatively small size of the vein. The easiest site is the femoral vein; however, the area needs to be kept clean after insertion, which can be difficult in infants. The next best site is the external jugular vein. Cannulation of this vein can be difficult because of the small size of the infant neck, but the vein can be visually located, which aids in insertion. The internal jugular vein is an excellent location for central vein access. The subclavian vein should be AVOIDED

Table 13-2. EMERGENCY MEDICATIONS IN PEDIATRIC PATIENTS

Medication	Dose	Indications	Precautions
*Atropine**	0.02 mg/kg Maximum doses: child—1 mg adolescent—2 mg	Bradycardia	Do not give <0.1 mg to prevent paradoxical bradycardia
Bretylium tosylate	5–10 mg/kg	Ventricular dysrhythmias refractory to lidocaine, procainamide	May cause hypotension; not recommended as infusion owing to long half-life
*Calcium chloride**	10 mg/kg	Hypocalcemia; hyperkalemia, hypermagnesemia	Same as for adults; no longer recommended for EMD or asystole
*Epinephrine**	0.02 mg/kg	Bradycardia	Same as for adults
Furosemide	1–2 mg/kg	Pulmonary/cerebral edema; fluid overload	May cause hypokalemia; dysrhythmias
Lidocaine	1 mg/kg	Same as for adults	Decrease dose by 50% for hepatic failure
Sodium Bicarbonate	$\dfrac{wt\ (kg)\ \times\ BD\dagger\ \times\ 0.3}{2}$	Same as for adults	Administer 4.2% (0.5 meq/cc) for infants <5 kg or <3 months of age
	NOTE: DO NOT ADMINISTER WITHOUT EFFECTIVE VENTILATION.		
Verapamil	0.1 mg/kg	Paroxysmal supraventricular tachycardia	May cause ↓ BP, CV collapse; use with caution for LV failure. Do not use in infants <1 yr

*NOTE: Overdose errors by a factor of 10 are frequently seen; caution is indicated to avoid this problem.
†BD = base deficit.

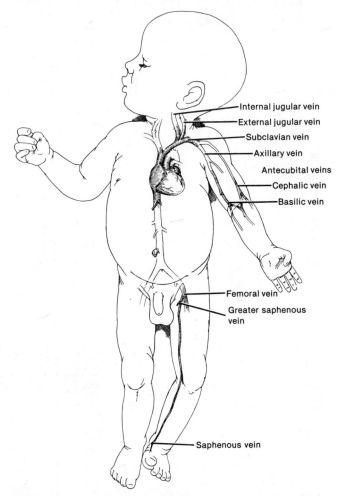

Figure 13–3. Locations of peripheral veins used for introduction of catheters. (Reproduced by permission from Levin DL et al (eds): A Practical Guide to Pediatric Intensive Care, 2nd ed. St. Louis, The CV Mosby Co., 1984.)

entirely in this age group, unless a pediatric surgeon or pediatric anesthesiologist is placing the catheter. The lung is very close to this vein and can be easily punctured. Also, if the subclavian artery is lacerated, it is extremely difficult to obtain hemostasis, owing to the location of the artery in relationship to the small size of the chest.

2. 6 Months–2 Years. The most accessible site is the femoral vein, followed by the external or internal jugular vein. The sub-clavian vein should be AVOIDED entirely.

3. 2–8 Years. Optimal sites and precautions are the same as for the previous age group.

4. 8 Years and Older. The sites are the same as for adults. The subclavian vein may be used in this age group, as the benefits of the line outweigh the risks involved in placement.

Miscellaneous Access

Types

1. Cutdown Saphenous/Femoral Lines. Peripheral vasoconstriction is commonly seen in hypovolemic and late septic (vasogenic) shock. Consequently, peripheral access can be extremely difficult. Often the only choice is to perform a cutdown to the saphenous vein. A large-bore catheter should be inserted to obtain optimal access. The length of the catheter should be short for the purpose of fluid resuscitation, but long for the patient who needs relatively little fluid resuscitation but is in need of vasopressor infusion and/or medication infusions. The femoral vein can also be used as a cutdown site.

2. Intraosseous Line. This procedure was widely used in infants and young children during the 1940s and 1950s, but after the introduction of plastic catheters for intravenous access, intraosseous infusion fell out of favor. It is becoming recognized once again, however, as a quick and efficient method of obtaining "intravenous" access in the infant or small child in shock. The bone marrow can be looked upon as a noncollapsible vein that is easily accessible and readily available.

A short bone marrow needle or spinal needle is used to cannulate the marrow (Fig. 13–4). Sites for cannulation include the tibia, distal femur, and iliac crest. Sternal puncture is not recommended in children, as the marrow is not as well developed as in the other sites, and the risk of puncturing the heart and other major organs is too great.

The needle to be used must have a solid stylet, to avoid obtaining a bone plug when the needle is introduced. When a "give" is felt, the stylet is removed, a syringe is placed at the end of the needle, and the marrow is aspirated. There must be marrow-blood return to demonstrate that the needle is in the correct location. The IV solution to be used is then connected to the needle as in any other IV setup. In the younger child, it is recommended that that IV solution have a "power" source behind it, to overcome the pressure in the marrow and aid in rapid infusion if desired. Blood pump bags or an infusion pump may be used. All medications and fluids can be infused via an intraosseous line. Cases of osteomyelitis occuring with this type of infusion have been reported, but it is a relatively rare complication.

1. Restrain limb, if necessary.
2. Position child in supine position.
3. Cleanse skin with povidone-iodine solution.
4. Locate site approximately 1.5–3 cm below and slightly medial to tibial tuberosity over flat edge of the bone.
5. Using aseptic technique, direct needle in a perpendicular or slightly inferior direction into bone marrow, avoiding epiphyseal plate.
6. Needle is in correct position when all the following conditions are present:
    a. There is a decrease in resistance after passing through the bone cortex.
    b. The needle is firmly in position and stands upright without support.
    c. Syringe aspiration yields bone marrow.
    d. There is a free flow of fluids with no significant subcutaneous infiltration.
7. Connect T-piece adapter and stopcock to needle.
8. Attach stopcock to appropriate IV infusion.
9. Stabilize needle on both sides with 2 × 2 inch gauze. Secure with tape, minimizing direct tension on needle.

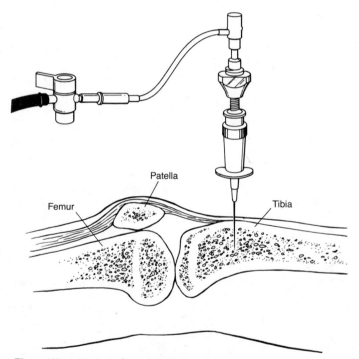

Patella

Femur

Tibia

Figure 13–4. Technique for intraosseous infusions: Intraosseous infusion in children can provide lifesaving therapy, but it is not without complications. The risk of intraosseous placement must be weighed against the benefit.

An intraosseous line should be used for short-term access only. When the child has been resuscitated, peripheral and/or central IV access should be easier to obtain. The intraosseous line is easy to place, with little training required to learn the technique, and it may be used in the prehospital setting with ease.

Helpful Hints

1. The pediatric trauma victim will need fluids administered, for which two large-bore peripheral IVs are optimal. Stopcocks should not be placed in line for a trauma victim, as they are 20-gauge in size, and the benefit of an 18-gauge catheter would be obliterated. "Short, fat lines" (large-gauge) will infuse the most fluid; "long, skinny lines" (small-gauge) will infuse the least.

2. The use of metrisets is mandatory for those under 1 year of age, since otherwise it is far too easy to infuse a large amount of fluid in a short amount of time in a small patient. Metrisets should be used on all pediatric patients for medication infusions. If the young patient needs a fluid challenge, it is often easier to push the fluid via a syringe rather than risk infusing the entire bag because someone wasn't watching the line.

3. NEVER hang a liter bag of fluid on patients less than 5 years of age in a code situation. People are too busy to watch the infusion, and the entire bag can be infused before anyone notices.

4. The fluid of choice in a trauma resuscitation is normal saline or lactated Ringer's solution—NEVER plain D5W. Isotonic fluids or blood is given to compensate for the estimated fluid loss. Dextrose can be added to the bag at a later time. Infants (<6 months) can become hypoglycemic during cardiac arrest, and the serum glucose level should be closely monitored. Often the patient will become hyperglycemic from the stress response of the body.

Lactated Ringer's or normal saline solution should also be used in resuscitation of the pediatric medical (non-trauma) patient. Medication infusions can be administered in plain D5W. It is important to watch the amount of "free water" infused, as damaged cells may swell with the excess free water, producing potential problems. A post-arrest problem may be cerebral edema due to excess D5W.

The exception to the "rule" is the patient with Reye's syndrome. These patients become hypoglycemic very quickly and often require D10W ½NS for maintenance fluid therapy (given at ⅔ maintenance rates). If the patient with Reye's syndrome suffers an arrest, it is most likely a respiratory arrest secondary to brain stem herniation.

EMERGENCY MEDICATIONS

As extensive coverage on cardiovascular pharmacology has already been provided in Chapter 9, our purpose here will be to

Table 13–3. MEDICATIONS DELIVERED BY INFUSION (Pediatric Variations)

Drug	Dose	Indications	Precautions
Dobutamine*	1–15 mcg/kg/min	Cardiogenic shock or low CO states	May cause tachycardia
Dopamine	10–20 mcg/kg/min (for vasopressor response)	Hypotension, vasogenic shock	Doses >25 mcg/kg/min not recommended, owing to vasoconstriction
Isuprel†	0.1–1.0 mcg/kg/min	Pacemaker failure; status asthmaticus	Same as for adult
Levophed & Regitine	5–40 cc/hr ("4:40")	Hypotension	Must be run via central vein. No untoward vasoconstriction with high doses
Lidocaine	20–40 mcg/kg/min	Same as for adults	Same as for adults
Nipride (nitroprusside)	1–10 mcg/kg/min	Same as for adults	Same as for adults

Preparation: 4 amps (16 mg) Levophed + 40 mg Regitine in 250 cc D5W = "4:40." Formula can be varied depending on degree of vasoconstriction or dilation required—for example, "2:40" would provide more beta effect, whereas "4:20" would provide more alpha effect. May concentrate to "16:160" and run wide open if necessary.

*Use "rule of 6s" (Table 13–4, #1) for preparation in D5W solution.
†Use modified "rule of 6s" (Table 13–4, #2) for preparation in D5W solution.

Table 13–4. "RULE OF 6s": MEDICATION INFUSION PREPARATION AND CALCULATION FOR PEDIATRIC PATIENTS

1. **"Rule of 6s":**
   A. 6 × wt in kg = mg to be added to 100 cc D5W
         OR
   B. 15 × wt in kg = mg to be added to 250 cc D5W
   C. Use with dopamine, dobutamine

       Above formulas yield: cc/hr = mcg/kg/min

   Example: To calculate for a 10-kg child to receive 8 mcg/kg/min of dopamine:

     6 × 10 = 60 mg dopamine to be added to 100 cc D5W
     Run at 8 cc/hr to deliver 8 mcg/kg/min
        OR
     15 × 10 = 150 mg dopamine to be added to 250 cc D5W
     Run at 8 cc/hr to deliver 8 mcg/kg/min

2. **"Modified" Rule of 6s:**
   A. 0.6 × wt in kg = mg to be added to 100 cc D5W
        OR
   B. 1.5 × wt in kg = mg to be added to 250 cc D5W
   C. Use with epinephrine, Isuprel

       Above formulas yield: 1 cc/hr = 0.1 mcg/kg/min

   D. 60 × wt in kg = mg to be added to 100 cc D5W
        OR
   E. 150 × wt in kg = mg to be added to 250 cc D5W
   F. Use with concentrated dopamine

       Above formulas yield: 1 cc/hr = 10 mcg/kg/min

3. **To determine cc/hr to be infused:**

$$cc/hr = \frac{\text{desired mcg/kg/min} \times 60 \text{ min/hr} \times \text{wt in kg}}{\text{mcg/cc}}$$

   Example: To calculate for a 15-kg child to receive a lidocaine infusion at 40 mcg/kg/min:

   1 g lidocaine in 250 cc D5W = 4000 mcg/cc

$$cc/hr = \frac{40 \text{ mcg/kg/min} \times 60 \text{ min/hr} \times \text{wt in kg}}{4000 \text{ mcg/cc}}$$

   $cc/hr = 9$

4. **To determine mcg/kg/min to be infused:**

$$mcg/kg/min = \frac{cc/hr \text{ being infused} \times \text{mcg/cc}}{\text{wt in kg} \times 60 \text{ min/hr}}$$

   Example: To calculate for the patient in the preceding example (15-kg child receiving lidocaine drip at 9 cc/hr):

$$\frac{9 \text{ cc/hr} \times 4000 \text{ mcg/cc}}{15 \text{ kg} \times 60 \text{ min/hr}} = 40 \text{ mcg/kg/min}$$

highlight pediatric variations with respect to dosage, indications, and precautions, as outlined in Tables 13–2, 13–3, 13–4.

Helpful Note on Medication Infusion:

When assembling IV tubing, it is helpful to place minimum-volume tubing in line for the pediatric patient. Anticipate having to give medications intravenously, and place a stopcock in line as close to the patient as possible (unless the patient is a trauma patient or the catheter is larger than 20-gauge). This will minimize the volume needed to flush emergency medications into the patient. Placement of a T-connector or extension tubing on the hub of the catheter will facilitate the transfer to different IV tubing setups, which commonly are changed when the patient is admitted or transported to another hospital.

REFERENCES

Benitz WE, Frankel LR, Stevenson DK: The pharmacology of neonatal resuscitation and cardiopulmonary intensive care. Part I. Immediate resuscitation. West J Med *144*:704, 1986; Part II. Extended intensive care. West J Med *145*:47, 1986.

Benson D, Benditt DG, Anderson RW: Cardiac arrest in young, ostensibly healthy patients: clinical, hemodynamic, and electrophysiologic findings. Am J Cardiol *52*:65, 1983.

Berg R: Emergency infusion of catecholamines into bone marrow. Am J Dis Child *138*:810, 1984.

Clinton J, McGill J, Irwin G: Cardiac arrest under age 40: etiology and prognosis. Ann Emerg Med *13*:1011, 1984.

Friedman WF, Fitzpatrick K, et al: The patent ductus arteriosus. Clin Perinatol *5*(2):411, 1978.

Friesen RM, Duncan P, Tweed WA, et al: Appraisal of pediatric cardiopulmonary resuscitation. CMA *12*:1055, 1982.

Heinild S, Sondergaard T, Tudvad F: Bone marrow infusion in childhood: experiences from a thousand infusions. J Pediatr *25*:1, 1944.

Hodge D: Intraosseous infusions: a review. Pediatr Emerg Care *1*:215, 1985.

Levin D, Morriss F, Moore G: A practical guide to pediatric intensive care. St. Louis, Mosby, 1984, Chapter 89.

Lewis J, Minter G, Eshelman SJ, et al: Outcome of pediatric resuscitation. Ann Emerg Med *12*:297, 1983.

Orlowski JP: Optimal position for external cardiac massage in infants and children. Crit Care Med *12*:224, 1984.

Orlowski JP: Pediatric cardiopulmonary resuscitation. Emerg Med Clin North Am *1*:3, 1983.

Orlowski JP: The effectiveness of pediatric cardiopulmonary resuscitation. Am J Dis Child *138*:1097, 1984.

Rosetti V, Thompson BM, Aprahamian C: Difficulty and delay in intravascular access in pediatric arrests. Ann Emerg Med *13*:406, 1984.

Suljaga-Pechtel K, Goldberg E, Strickon P: Cardiopulmonary resuscitation in a hospitalized population: prospective study of factors associated with outcome. Resuscitation *12*:77, 1984.

Trophy DE, Minter MG, Thompson B: Cardiorespiratory arrest and resuscitation of children. Am J Dis Child *138*:1099, 1984.

14

TRAUMATIC CARDIAC ARREST

GENERAL CONSIDERATIONS

The management of cardiac arrest due to trauma is different from that for arrest due to nontraumatic causes, since the etiology of the traumatic arrest is more likely to be severe hypovolemia, tension pneumothorax, or cardiac tamponade than myocardial dysfunction or primary arrhythmias. The ABCs of basic resuscitation must still be followed.

INITIAL THERAPY

A. If cervical spine injury is suspected, airway must be maintained with the jaw-lift technique, and intubation performed with the neck immobilized and under traction.

B. Tension pneumothorax must be searched for and immediately treated by inserting a 14-gauge needle into the 2nd anterior intercostal space of the affected side. Tube thoracostomy can be performed later, after the patient is successfully resuscitated.

C. Immediate thoracotomy must be performed to relieve possible cardiac tamponade and allow direct cardiac compression (open-chest massage), if tension pneumothorax is absent or its decompression does not resuscitate the patient. External chest compression is ineffective in the presence of severe hypovolemia or cardiac tamponade. Emergency thoracotomy will also allow control of bleeding from the great vessels, temporary repair of myocardial wounds, and cross-clamping of the aorta to control intra-abdominal hemorrhage until definitive repair is possible.

Emergency Thoracotomy Procedure (See Table 14–1 for needed minimal supplies):

1. In the emergent situation, time should not be wasted on chest preparation or sterile technique.
2. Make an incision below the nipple in the male, or along the breast fold in the female (approximately 4th intercostal space), from the sternal border to the posterior axillary line down to the intercostal muscle.
3. Divide the intercostal muscle and, while temporarily stopping ventilation to collapse the lungs, puncture the pleura. Cut the intercostal muscle along the top of the 5th rib (see Fig. 14–1).

Table 14–1. EMERGENCY THORACOTOMY: EQUIPMENT AND SUPPLIES

	Have readily available:
1. No. 20 scalpel with handle	1. Defibrillator with internal paddles
2. Mayo scissors	2. Chest tube
3. Rib spreader	3. Autotransfusion set-up
4. Forceps (10-inch)	4. Suction device
5. Vascular clamps	5. Teflon patches
6. 2-0 silk sutures with curved blunt needle	6. Foley catheter (20F, 30 ml balloon) to tamponade stellate wounds
7. Suture scissors	

4. Insert the rib retractor. The ribs above and below the incision can be cut at the costochondral junction to improve access.

5. If the myocardium cannot be evaluated through the pericardium, open the pericardium longitudinally on the anterolateral surface, using Mayo scissors held parallel

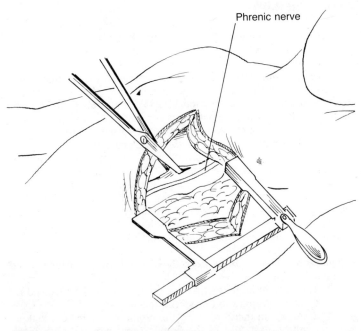

Phrenic nerve

Figure 14–1. Left anterolateral thoracotomy. An incision is made between the fourth and fifth interspaces. It is important to stay as close to the top of the fifth rib as possible to avoid the intercostal artery. The rib spreader should be placed with the handle down. Pericardiotomy is started near the diaphragm and anterior to the phrenic nerve. (Reproduced with permission from Roberts JR, Hedges JR: Clinical Procedures in Emergency Medicine. Philadelphia, WB Saunders, 1985, p. 253.)

to the surface of the heart with just the tip penetrating the pericardium. Avoid the phrenic nerve.

6. Quickly remove any clots with a sweeping motion of the fingers.

7. If spontaneous contractions are absent, perform open cardiac compression by squeezing the heart between the palmar surfaces of all the fingers of both hands. Do not use just fingertip pressure. Avoid compression of the coronary arteries.

8. Compress at a rate of 80 per minute.

9. Repair or occlude any cardiac wounds.

10. Inspect the great vessels for any injury, and compress or clamp as necessary.

11. If intra-abdominal hemorrhaging is suspected, bluntly dissect the descending aorta free from the pleura and esophagus, and cross-clamp with digital pressure or use a vascular clamp. The aorta should not be occluded for longer than 30–60 minutes and can be unclamped for 30–60 seconds every 10 minutes to allow for renal and spinal cord perfusion.

12. To defibrillate, internal cardiac paddles should be placed over the right and left ventricles and discharged using 20 joules of energy. Repeat as needed at the same energy setting, since higher energy can cause myocardial necrosis. NOTE: If internal paddles are unavailable, pediatric paddles can be used as a last resort.

13. The epicardium should be kept moist with normal saline.

D. Multiple large-bore (≥16 gauge) IV lines should be inserted either percutaneously or via cutdown, and 2–3 liters of crystalloid solution (normal saline, lactated Ringer's) infused rapidly. Internal jugular or subclavian lines should be avoided because of the increased difficulty for insertion and greater risk of injury to the vessels in their collapsed state. Antecubital, saphenous, or femoral vein cannulation is preferred. Type-specific or universal donor blood (O negative) should be infused if hypovolemia persists after 3 liters of crystalloid solution have been given. Blood from the thoracic cavity can be autotransfused.

E. Pneumatic devices such as MAST (Military or Medical Antishock Trousers) should be applied and inflated if continued bleeding below the diaphragm is suspected. These devices contain three independently inflatable chambers, one in each leg and one in the abdominal flap (see Fig. 14–2). Pneumatic devices provide circulatory support by (1) increasing peripheral vascular resistance, thereby directing the effective circulatory volume to the essential organs (heart, brain, and lungs); (2) increasing intra-abdominal pressure and indirectly tamponading intra-abdominal bleeding; and (3) direct tamponade of major limb vessels.

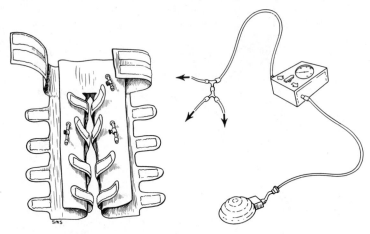

Figure 14–2. MAST suit is inflatable three-compartment garment. (Reproduced with permission from Moore EE, Eiseman B, Van Way CW III: Critical Decisions in Trauma. St. Louis, CV Mosby, 1984, p. 558.)

MAST Application (Figs. 14–3 to 14–8)
1. Open the trousers fully and place the patient onto the trousers while maintaining spine immobilization if indi-

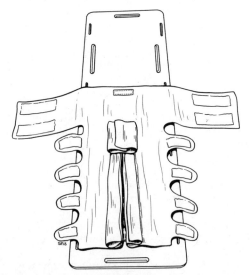

Figure 14–3. MAST suit should be placed on stretcher before patient is positioned. (Reproduced with permission from Moore EE, Eiseman B, Van Way CW III: Critical Decisions in Trauma. St. Louis, CV Mosby, 1984, p. 559.)

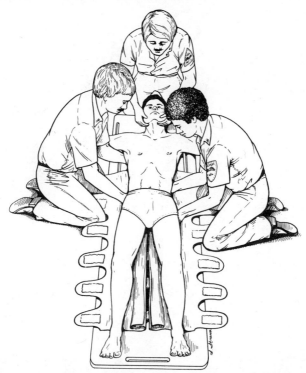

Figure 14–4. Optimally, clothes should be removed to facilitate rapid perusal of patient before MAST is fastened. (Reproduced with permission from Moore EE, Eiseman B, Van Way CW III: *Critical Decisions in Trauma*. St. Louis, CV Mosby, 1984, p. 559.)

cated. The patient should be as fully undressed as possible below the waist.

2. Wrap the legs and abdomen snugly and fasten the Velcro binders.

3. Attach the foot pump hoses to the tubing of each chamber. *Optional*: Prime the chambers by blowing into the tubing prior to connecting the foot pump.

4. A stopcock on the tubing of each chamber controls the sequence of inflation. Open the stopcock of the chamber to be inflated, while keeping the others closed. Always inflate the injured leg first, to avoid exacerbating any bleeding. *Inflate the abdominal compartment last*.

5. Inflate until compartment pressure is 100 mm Hg (in models with gauges) or until the pop-off valve pops. Lower inflation pressures are less effective. Close the stopcock when the chamber is inflated.

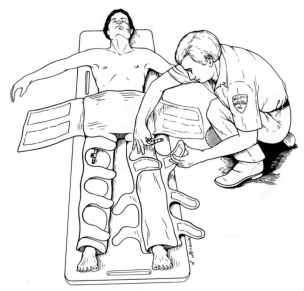

Figure 14–5. Velcro fasteners should be closed tightly. (Reproduced with permission from Moore EE, Eiseman B, Van Way CW III: Critical Decisions in Trauma. St. Louis, CV Mosby, 1984, p. 560.)

6. Check compartment pressures frequently, especially during environmental temperature or altitude changes, and maintain full inflation.

7. Monitor vital signs every 5 minutes while pants are inflated.

8. Never remove or deflate MAST suddenly without adequate means of maintaining blood pressure support, since irreversible shock may ensue.

9. When indicated, deflate pants slowly, beginning with the abdominal chamber, then the uninjured leg, and, lastly, the injured leg. Stop deflation whenever systolic blood pressure drops more than 5 mm Hg. Continue deflation after blood pressure is restored.

10. When deflating, arterial blood gas measurements must be closely monitored to detect and treat metabolic acidosis caused by prolonged ischemia of the areas covered by the trousers.

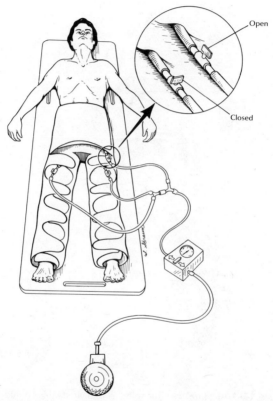

Figure 14–6. Tubing is connected to all three compartments. Insert illustrates closed and open positions for valves. (Reproduced with permission from Moore EE, Eiseman B, Van Way CW III: Critical Decisions in Trauma. St. Louis, CV Mosby, 1984, p. 560.)

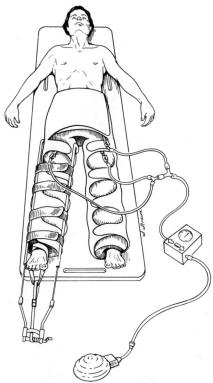

Figure 14–7. If Hare traction splint is indicated, this should be placed before MAST is inflated. (Reproduced with permission from Moore EE, Eiseman B, Van Way CW III: Critical Decisions in Trauma. St. Louis, CV Mosby, 1984, p. 561.)

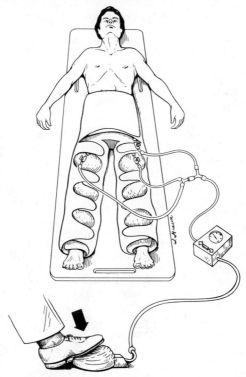

Figure 14–8. Position of valves to each compartment must be checked before inflation. Leg sections should be inflated first. (Reproduced with permission from Moore EE, Eiseman B, Van Way CW III: Critical Decisions in Trauma. St. Louis, CV Mosby, 1984, p. 561.)

OUTCOME

Survival following emergency thoracotomy for traumatic cardiac arrest depends on the mechanism of injury (blunt vs. penetrating), duration of arrest (at scene vs. in ED), and response to thoracotomy and cross-clamping. Cardiac arrest due to blunt trauma is associated with poor long-term survival (<3%). In contrast, arrest due to penetrating trauma is associated with 30–40% survival, higher for low-velocity wounds (e.g., knife wound) than for high-velocity wounds (e.g., gunshot). Failure to maintain systolic blood pressure above 70 mm Hg despite aggressive management is invariably associated with a fatal outcome.

NEAR–DROWNING

DEFINITIONS

1. *Drowning* is defined as death by suffocation in water.
2. *Near-drowning* implies that survival has occurred at least temporarily following submersion.
3. Drowning and near-drowning episodes may be further defined as being with or without aspiration, the latter referring to hypoxia and suffocation as a result of laryngospasm but without aspiration of water. Between 10% and 15% of drownings occur without aspiration.
4. Other terms used include:
    a. *Secondary drowning* (also known as delayed drowning, or post-immersion syndrome), defined as a near-drowning episode followed by recurrence of respiratory symptoms and death minutes to days after the initial episode.
    b. *Immersion syndrome*, referring to sudden death following submersion in cold water (probably a result of arrhythmias induced by vagal stimulation).

INCIDENCE

Drowning accounts for approximately 9000 deaths annually in the United States and is the third leading cause of accidental deaths. The greatest incidence is in the second decade, and in individuals under the age of 4. The incidence of near-drowning may be as high as 80,000 per year.

Cases of children surviving after prolonged immersion (up to 40 minutes) in cold water have been reported.

CLINICAL PRESENTATION

1. The major consequences of near-drowning are hypoxia, acidosis, and pulmonary edema.
2. Acidosis (combined respiratory and metabolic) invariably follows near-drowning episodes. Often by the time a victim reaches the emergency department (following spontaneous breathing or external ventilation), the Pco_2 is normal and the pH is low, indicating that the respiratory acidosis has been corrected and the metabolic acidosis (caused by lactic acid) remains.

3. Pulmonary edema occurs in up to 75% of near-drowning cases.

4. Significant electrolyte abnormalities are usually not present in near-drowning.

5. The hematocrit is usually normal, although hemolysis can occur (seen more with freshwater near-drownings).

6. Renal abnormalities, including renal failure, have been reported. These are perhaps a result of hypotension and lactic acidosis, although other causes, such as myglobinuria, should be considered.

7. Differences in the tonicity of salt- and freshwater, while theoretically likely to cause differences pathophysiologically, for all practical purposes result in a similar clinical picture for patients who survive near-drowning episodes.

8. Drowning may be a complication of another condition. For example, cervical spinal cord injury may occur as a result of a diving accident, leading to near-drowning. Alcohol and drug intoxication may be the primary cause. Hypothermia, seizures, hypoglycemia, air embolus (for example, in scuba divers), and nonaccidental drownings (suicide, homicide, child abuse) may be associated with near-drowning episodes.

INITIAL TREATMENT (PREHOSPITAL)

In general, attempts to drain water from the lungs are time-wasting efforts. In freshwater near-drownings, most of the water is rapidly absorbed through the alveoli. The situation with seawater near-drownings is slightly different, and water may be present in the alveoli. Maintaining the patient in a head-down, feet-up position (Trendelenburg position) will result in sufficient gravity drainage to allow available water to drain.

Mouth-to-mouth resuscitation (to be started in the water if necessary) and chest compression (to be started once the patient is removed from the water) must be initiated if spontaneous respiration and/or pulse is absent. There should be a thorough effort to locate a pulse; this may be difficult owing to peripheral vasoconstriction and low cardiac output.

Consider associated injuries, such as cervical spine injury, which should be stabilized with a collar, backboard, and sandbags. Upper airway obstruction (for example, by seaweed, sand, or other particulate matter), should be removed manually, if possible, or with a Heimlich maneuver. If mouth-to-mouth ventilation is unsuccessful, airway obstruction should be suspected and a Heimlich maneuver performed. However, when there is no evidence of foreign body airway obstruction, the routine use of a Heimlich maneuver is not recommended as part of the initial management of drowning victims.

Table 15–1. MANAGEMENT OF NEAR-DROWNING IN THE EMERGENCY DEPARTMENT

1. Airway management:
     Unconscious—endotracheal intubation
     Stuporous—endotracheal intubation
     Alert—mask or nasal cannula
2. Hyperventilation with oxygen in as high a concentration as possible
3. ECG monitor
4. Intravenous line—keep open rate with normal saline
5. Rewarming of hypothermic patients
6. Laboratory tests:
     Arterial blood gases
     Hematocrit, white blood count
     Electrolytes
7. Nasogastric tube (for serious episodes or in intubated patients)
8. Foley catheter (for serious episodes)

PREHOSPITAL ADVANCED LIFE SUPPORT PROCEDURES

Establishment of an adequate airway is the highest priority. Endotracheal intubation is preferred if available. Patient should receive 100% oxygen. Non-intubated patients should receive oxygen through a non-rebreathing mask in as high a concentration as possible. Control of the airway is particularly important, as copious secretions and regurgitated fluids may obstruct the airway.

Start an IV line with lactated Ringer's or normal saline solution. In general, volume support is not a critical aspect of therapy, and infusion should initially be at a "keep-open" rate.

Cardiac monitoring is important, as hypoxia and acidosis may result in arrhythmias.

Because of the invariable acidosis, some physicians recommend empiric administration of sodium bicarbonate (0.5–1.0 mEq/kg) for well-documented near-drowning episodes.

Core temperature may be lowered as a result of cold-water immersions. Thus, efforts to maintain and elevate body temperature should be initiated. In a prehospital setting, this is usually confined to the use of blankets and heated vehicles.

EMERGENCY DEPARTMENT PROCEDURES

Airway management deserves top priority in the emergency department. If not already accomplished, endotracheal intubation should be performed in the stuporous or unconscious patient (see Table 15–1).

Patients should be hyperventilated, with oxygen administered in as high a concentration as possible initially. For mild near-drowning episodes this may merely require a nasal cannula; for more serious episodes, non-rebreathing masks with continuous positive airway pressure (CPAP) and/or endotracheal intubation with positive end-expiratory pressure (PEEP) may be required.

Obtain blood gases, hematocrit, white blood count, and serum electrolytes. Patients should be on an ECG monitor. A gastric tube is indicated to decompress the stomach of aspirated water or of air aspirated as a result of CPR. A Foley catheter should be inserted and urinary output monitored.

A 12-lead cardiogram is especially important in elderly patients or individuals with underlying heart disease, in order to detect myocardial infarction, ischemia, or arrhythmias.

Bronchospasm should be managed with IV aminophylline or inhaled terbutaline or Bronkosol.

Cardiac arrhythmias are often the result of hypoxia, hypothermia, or acidosis, and correction of these conditions will frequently abolish the rhythm disturbance.

Patients with apparent mild near-drowning episodes should be closely observed for at least 24 hours. Post-immersion syndrome may occur in individuals who appear to have recovered from a near-drowning episode. Respiratory symptoms usually begin within several hours, and may be profound. Therefore, admission for observation is usually warranted in near-drowning episodes.

PROGNOSIS

The prognosis for drowning patients requiring CPR correlates with the level of consciousness following resuscitation. Conn and colleagues categorize patients as A (awake), B (blunted), or C (comatose) following successful CPR. Patients in category A have 100% survival, with excellent neurologic recovery. Patients in category C have a survival rate of 82%, with only half becoming neurologically normal.

REFERENCES

Conn AW, Barker GA: Fresh water drowning and neardrowning—an update. Can Anaesth Soc J *31*:s38, 1984.

Conn AW, Montes JE, Barker GA, et al: Cerebral salvage in neardrowning following neurological classification by triage. Can Anaesth Soc J *27*:201, 1980.

Frewen TC, Sumabat WO, Han VK, et al: Cerebral resuscitation therapy in pediatric neardrowning. J Pediatr *106*:615, 1985.

Knopp R: Near drowning. JACEP *7*:249, 1978.

Modell JH: Drown versus near-drown: A discussion of definitions. Crit Care Med *9*:351, 1981.

Modell JH, Graves AS, Kuck EJ: Neardrowning: Correlation of level of consciousness and survival. Can Anaesth Soc J *27*:211, 1980.

Moser RH: Drowning: a seasonal disease. JAMA *229*:563, 1974.

Neal JM: Near-drowning. J Emerg Med *3*:41, 1985.

Ornato J: The resuscitation of near-drowning victims. JAMA *256*:75, 1986.

Pearn J: Pathophysiology of drowning. Med J Australia *142*:586, 1985.

16

HYPOTHERMIA

DEFINITION AND ETIOLOGY

Hypothermia is defined as a core body temperature below 35°C (95°F). Because many standard medical thermometers do not read below 34.4°C, clinical hypothermia can be easily overlooked.

Most clinically significant episodes of hypothermia result from an accidental fall in core body temperature due to injury, immersion in cold water, or prolonged exposure to a cold environment. The very young and the very old are the most susceptible. Infants lose the same amount of heat per unit area as adults but cannot produce as much heat. Older individuals are more susceptible than the young to environmental cold, owing to a lower metabolic rate.

Alcohol ingestion increases the risk of hypothermia by causing cutaneous vasodilation, impairment of the shivering mechanism, hypothalamic dysfunction, and a lack of awareness of the environment.

Other medical conditions associated with the development of accidental hypothermia include drug ingestion (especially barbiturates or phenothiazines), diabetes (especially in the presence of hypoglycemia), hypothyroidism, hypopituitarism, hypoadrenalism, anorexia nervosa, head injury, and sepsis.

Immersion in cold water is more serious than exposure to cold air, because cold water has 32 times greater thermal conductivity than air.

Hypothermia can occur in previously healthy individuals (such as cross-country skiers or hikers) who become injured and are exposed to the cold for prolonged periods.

CLINICAL FEATURES

Reflex vasoconstriction helps to preserve the core temperature, but makes detection of the pulse and blood pressure difficult. The hypothermic patient may appear clinically dead but may still be viable with proper diagnosis and aggressive management. Successful clinical recovery has occurred in a patient with an initial core temperature as low as 17°C.

Mild degrees of hypothermia (above 30°C) result in shivering, loss of fine motor coordination, and lethargy. At core body temperatures below 30° C, the pupils usually dilate and hyporeflexia occurs. When body temperature falls below 20°C, the electroencephalogram may be flat.

Hemodynamically, mild hypothermia causes a rise in pulse rate, blood pressure, peripheral vascular resistance, central venous pressure, and cardiac output. Moderate to severe hypothermia (below 30°C) causes bradycardia, arrhythmias (atrial fibrillation is common, but other atrial, junctional, or ventricular arrhythmias can occur), hypotension, and a fall in cardiac output. The risk of ventricular fibrillation or asystole increases as the temperature drops below 28°C. The J wave (Osborn wave), shown below, which is most prominent in leads V3 or V4, occurs in 80% of hypothermia patients and increases in size with decreasing core body temperature.

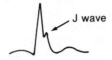

Oxygenation and acid-base balance are altered by hypothermia. Mild hypothermia initially causes hyperventilation. As core temperature decreases respiratory depression occurs. A combined respiratory and metabolic acidosis may occur as a result of hypoventilation, carbon dioxide retention, poor peripheral perfusion, and increased lactic acid production.

Other effects of hypothermia include: (1) diuresis and volume depletion due to inhibition of the release of antidiuretic hormone; (2) elevated hematocrit due to dehydration and splenic contraction; (3) increase in plasma viscosity (especially at temperatures below 27°C); and (4) hyperglycemia due to inhibition of insulin release. The hyperglycemia reverts with rewarming and usually does not require treatment with insulin.

TREATMENT

General Principles

Early recognition of hypothermia is important. Maintain a high index of suspicion in any patient with an altered level of consciousness who has been subjected to even a modestly cool environment. A thermometer (rectal or probe) capable of registering a temperature of 30° C or less is essential.

The hypothermic heart is susceptible to serious arrhythmias, and care should be taken to move the patient gently during transportation or during transfer from a litter to a hospital bed. The ECG rhythm should be monitored continuously.

Routine laboratory evaluation usually includes arterial blood gases, complete blood count, prothrombin time, partial thrombo-plastin time, glucose, electrolytes, blood urea nitrogen, serum creatinine, amylase, liver function tests, electrocardiogram, chest x-ray, and urinalysis.

The hypothermic heart is usually unresponsive to cardioactive drugs, pacemaker stimulation, and defibrillation, and these inter-ventions are generally not useful until the core temperature is increased to above 30°C. Endotracheal intubation of the severely hypothermic patient may be needed in order to protect the airway, to correct hypoxemia and hypercarbia, and to deliver warm hu-midified oxygen. Intubation is unlikely to precipitate ventricular fibrillation, provided the patient is adequately ventilated (usually with a bag-valve-mask device) and acidosis is corrected prior to intubation.

The effect of most drugs and hormones is diminished during hypothermia. In addition, metabolism of drugs and hormones is usually reduced, causing accumulation in the body and potential toxicity during rewarming if repeated doses have been adminis-tered. Nonessential drugs and hormones should generally be avoided until the temperature is above 30°C. Hypoglycemia should be treated with glucose. Hyperglycemia during hypothermia will often correct spontaneously with rewarming; the use of insulin may be necessary in specific cases, but there is the hazard that this may induce hypoglycemia as the body tempeature is corrected. Volume depletion should be corrected.

Prehospital Management

Every effort should be made to minimize further heat loss, to begin the rewarming process, and to cautiously transport the patient to the hospital. If possible, wet garments should be removed and replaced with dry (preferably warm) garments. Blankets and/or an insulated sleeping bag may be used to retain body heat. A normo-thermic rescuer may lie alongside the victim underneath the covers to assist in rewarming. Airway rewarming with warm humidified oxygen, if available, should be done.

Mild to Moderate Hypothermia (≥30° C)

Patients with mild to moderate hypothermia (30°C or above) generally have a good prognosis regardless of the rewarming method used. External rewarming is most appropriate, either passively, using blankets and allowing the patient's own metabolism to restore normothermia, or actively, by means of electric blankets, hot water bottles, or warm baths. Although effective, warm baths have the disadvantage of not allowing the cardiac rhythm to be monitored. If hypothermia has developed over a prolonged period of time, the core temperature should probably be restored gradually (at a rate of 0.5–1.0°C per hour).

Severe Hypothermia (<30°C)

In severely hypothermic patients, attempts at rewarming by application of external heat (such as immersion of the patient in a warm water bath) are hazardous, because sudden peripheral vasodilation will cause perfusion of vascular beds containing cold, lactic acid–rich blood. Return of this blood into the central core may cause a temporary paradoxical "after-drop" in core temperature and pH, increasing the likelihood of ventricular fibrillation. For this reason, patients with severe hypothermia should generally be treated with core rewarming. The most popular current techniques include: (1) administration of warmed intravenous fluids through a central line; (2) warm (42–46°C) humidified oxygen (most effective by endotracheal tube); (3) peritoneal lavage using a fluid temperature of 43°C; and (4) mediastinal irrigation and cardiopulmonary bypass (usually reserved for severe hypothermia complicated by cardiac arrest).

Hypothermia-Induced Cardiac Arrest

Treatment of a patient in cardiac arrest due to hypothermia is different from treatment of a normothermic patient in cardiac arrest. The most common cardiac rhythm in hypothermia-induced arrest is ventricular fibrillation or asystole. However, the fibrillating hypothermic heart is often resistant to defibrillation until the core temperature is raised. The temperature at which the hypothermic fibrillation heart will respond to defibrillation is variable. In general, defibrillation should be attempted as soon as possible. If unsuccessful, CPR should be continued and aggressive attempts should be made to rapidly rewarm the core, using a combination of techniques (including cardiopulmonary bypass and peritoneal lavage), with repeated attempts at defibrillation periodically as the core temperature increases. The patient should be intubated as soon as possible.

The decision to terminate resuscitation is based on the unique circumstances of each incident. In general, children or young adults who develop cardiac arrest owing to a sudden severe drop in core temperature (as in cold water immersion) should be treated aggressively, since survival without neurologic impairment may be possible.

REFERENCES

Carden D, Doan L, Sweeney PJ, et al: Hypothermia (clinical conference). Ann Emerg Med *11*:408, 1982.

Fitzgerald FT, Jessop C: Accidental hypothermia: a report of 22 cases and review of the literature. In Stollerman GH (ed): Advances in Internal Medicine, Vol 27. Chicago, Year Book, 1982, pp 127–150.

Kurtz KJ: Hypothermia in the elderly: the cold facts. Geriatrics *37*:85, 1982.

Reuler JB: Hypothermia: pathophysiology, clinical settings, and management. Ann Intern Med *89*:519, 1978.

White JD: Hypothermia: the Bellevue experience. Ann Emerg Med *11*:417, 1982.

Wong KC: Physiology and pharmacology of hypothermia. West J Med *138*:227, 1983.

Zell SC, Kurtz KJ: Severe exposure hypothermia: a resuscitation protocol. Ann Emerg Med *14*:339, 1985.

17

LEGAL CONSIDERATIONS

INTRODUCTION

The decision to initiate or withhold CPR is a legal as well as a medical problem that must be faced by health care providers as each case arises. Patient and family preferences and quality of life considerations are increasingly being factored into the decision-making process. Nevertheless, the physician in charge of the patient is ultimately responsible for the final decision. This chapter presents guidelines to help the clinician make a decision in any individual case.

Clinicians and others responsible for the administration of advanced cardiac life support (ACLS) should be aware of the existing laws within the state in which they practice. These are established either by the legislature passing a law relevant to cardiac resuscitation, withdrawal of life-sustaining treatment, declaring an individual dead, and so forth (known as legislative law), or by cases decided in the appellate or state supreme court (known as case law). Cases that are decided at the entry level courts and not appealed to higher courts generally do not supply a precedent for case law.

A full discussion of all the legal issues surrounding cardiopulmonary resuscitation is beyond the scope of this manual, but critical questions raised about CPR and legal matters are discussed. The following section presents questions foremost in the minds of clinicians managing critically ill patients.

LEGAL QUESTIONS IN CRITICAL CARE

1. When Should CPR Be Initiated?

Emergency medical technicians and paramedics in the prehospital setting and physicians and nurses in the hospital setting are obligated to initiate CPR in any situation in which the patient's brain is potentially viable and there are no immediately known medical or legal contraindications to resuscitating the patient. Except in cases in which death is obviously irreversible (decapitation, presence of rigor mortis, or dependent lividity), the brain must be assumed to be potentially viable. Since it is impossible in most instances to determine whether the brain is potentially viable, legally one must assume that the brain is potentially viable. Therefore, the rule is: When in doubt, CPR should be initiated.

"NO-CODE" DOCUMENTATION POLICY

1. Every patient admitted is automatically placed in Code Status A (maximal therapeutic effort).

2. The consent of the patient or his/her legal representative is required to change the status of a patient to Code B or C (therapeutic measures withheld or withdrawn). The form "Authorization to Withhold or Limit Therapeutic Measures" must be filled out and placed in the physician's orders, and a note must be written in the patient's record documenting the change. A resident may write the order *after obtaining the concurrence of the patient's attending physician.* The attending physician must countersign the order within 24 hours.

3. A patient may be returned to code status "A" at any time, using the above procedure.

4. It is recognized that the "No-Code" policies contained herein cannot be completed in certain rapidly evolving emergent situations. In such emergencies, the responsible physician may need to make decisions changing code status without following all these procedures, in accord with his/her clinical judgment.

GUIDELINES FOR DOCUMENTING A CHANGE IN CODE STATUS

1. Why the patient is being designated a "No-Code." (The medical reason for the decision—include diagnosis and what diagnostic/therapeutic measures have been taken.)

2. Do you consider the patient competent to consent to decisions about his/her care? (Document the reasons.)

3. Has the patient or his/her family participated in this decision? (Document what was told the patient/family, what they said, who witnessed the conversation— the latter should be another member of the health care team.)

4. If the patient is not competent to make the decisions, obtain and document the following:

    a. Statements from two (2) physicians (not on the primary team) regarding *concurrence with the patient's prognosis and treatment plan.*

    b. The name of the legal next-of-kin or guardian who participated in the decision.

    c. What was told the kin/guardian, what they said, who witnessed the conversation (the latter should be another member of the health care team).

5. What therapeutic measures are to be withheld or discontinued?

Figure 17–1. Form outlining "No-Code" documentation policy. (Modified with permission from Loren C. Winterscheid, M.D., Medical Director, University Hospital, Seattle, WA.)

Illustration continued on opposite page

PHYSICIAN'S AUTHORIZATION TO WITHHOLD OR LIMIT
THERAPEUTIC MEASURES

PATIENT NAME	NO.	DATE

CODES: A: Maximal therapeutic effort

B: Selective limitation of therapeutic measures as specified below. All other measures may be given.

C: All life-maintaining measures can be discontinued. (Any measures indicated to ensure maximum patient comfort may be continued or instituted.)

CHANGE IN CODE STATUS:

FROM	TO

SPECIFIC MEASURES TO BE WITHHELD:

- ☐ cardiopulmonary resuscitation
- ☐ defibrillation/countershock
- ☐ mechanical ventilation
- ☐ endotracheal intubation
- ☐ intravenous vasoactive drugs
- ☐ antiarrhythmics
- ☐ oxygen therapy
- ☐ antibiotics
- ☐ invasive monitoring (Swan-Ganz catheter, central line, arterial line)
- ☐ other

Signature of Physician

Printed Name   Date   Signature of Attending Physician

Name of Attending Physician with Whom Discussed   Printed Name   Date

Figure 17–1 *Continued*

Ample case law supports the medical decision to support cardio-vascular and respiratory function before determination of brain viability can be made.

2. When Should CPR Be Withheld?

The only indications for withholding CPR are (a) when there is obvious indication of death (decapitation, rigor mortis, dependent lividity), and (b) when there is competent patient refusal to have CPR initiated. The length of time from collapse to initiation of CPR is not a valid reason to withhold CPR. In other words, one cannot assume that brain death has occurred because of delay in initiation of treatment. In may be argued that a low level of cardiac activity had been occurring up to and just before ACLS became available. Furthermore, it is impossible to get completely accurate data about the length of collapse prior to initiation of resuscitation. CPR may be withheld if there is competent patient refusal to have CPR initiated. Competent patient refusal may come about through a properly executed physician's directive or by durable power of attorney. Since it is unlikely in the prehospital situation or in the emergency department to have this information, one must assume that such competent patient refusal does not exist. In the in-hospital situation, however, such information may be available, often placed in the chart as a "Do Not Resuscitate" order by the physician.

3. When Are "Do Not Resuscitate" (DNR) Orders Appropriate?

"Do Not Resuscitate" orders are appropriate for situations in which there is an irreversible (no known cure), irreparable (disease has gone beyond the reparative state) condition in which death is imminent. Imminent is defined as "within 2 weeks." It is reasonable to infer that patients who have living wills specifically stating that there be no extraordinary life-sustaining measures may have "Do Not Resuscitate" orders written. In other situations, the "Do Not Resuscitate" order should be discussed with family members or legal guardians and documentation in the medical record placed summarizing the patient's decision, the patient's condition, and the decision to withhold CPR. These orders should be in writing and signed by the physician on the order sheet. An example of a "No Code" documentation policy is shown in Figure 17–1.

4. When Should CPR Be Terminated, Once Initiated?

CPR may be stopped when a doctor, either in person or via radio or telephone (in a supervisory medical control role), has certified the unresponsiveness of the patient to resuscitative procedures. Several articles and editorials have recommended that CPR be terminated after a period of 30–45 minutes in the face of cardiovascular unresponsiveness. The problem with using duration of resuscitation as a basis to terminate CPR is that, although the odds of success become increasingly remote with longer resuscitation attempts, there *have* been recoveries following exceedingly long resuscitation efforts. Furthermore, it is unreliable to conclude that permanent and irreversible brain damage may occur as a result of a long resuscitation. While the chances of a full neurologic recovery may be slight, instances have occurred.

For patients who have received basic and advanced cardiac life support but in whom maintenance of a spontaneous pulse and establishment of blood pressure have not been achieved after accepted efforts at resuscitation, the decision may be made to stop resuscitation. "Accepted measures of resuscitation" means specifically the protocols and guidelines put forth by the Heart Association and summarized in this manual. Thus, the only basis for termination of CPR is lack of cardiovascular responsiveness, and the duration of resuscitation must always be a judgment.

The issue of brain death is moot in the patient with cardiovascular unresponsiveness. Since the brain is far more sensitive to hypoxia than the heart, it is assumed that cardiovascular unresponsiveness entails brain death.

The decision of when to stop CPR can be based upon far more than the length of resuscitation. Other factors include the patient's age, temporary response to administered medications, medical history, family desires, and so on. In the final analysis, no formula or clock can tell a physician when to stop a resuscitation. The decision to stop resuscitative efforts will always be an agonizing decision.

5. When Should Life-Sustaining Systems Be Withdrawn?

For patients meeting brain death criteria, the decision is relatively easy. The President's Commission has formulated the *Uniform Determination of Death:*

"An individual who has sustained either irreversible cessation of circulatory and respiratory functions, or irreversible cessation of all functions of the entire brain, including the brain stem, is dead. A determination of death must be made in accordance with accepted medical standards." (See reference 1.)

This definition is slightly different from the Harvard criteria, which require absent spinal cord reflexes and two EEGs 24 hours apart (reference 2). Brain death criteria apply only in the absence of hypothermia, shock, or drug effects (for example, barbiturate overdose), metabolic derangements, or recent hypoxia. Since hypoxia is the inevitable result of cardiac arrest, and since it is impossible to quantitate the duration of hypoxia, not to mention the frequent presence of cardiogenic shock, it is difficult to know how much time should pass before the patient is declared brain dead. It seems reasonable to wait a minimum of 24 hours.

Cortical brain death is determined by EEG, radioisotope studies, or arteriography. Death of the brain stem is determined by the absence of pupillary function, spontaneous respirations, reflexively controlled eye movements, corneal reflexes, facial muscle movement, and pharyngeal movement. Brain stem death is not compatible with life, as spontaneous heart activity cannot be maintained.

The question of when to withdraw life-sustaining support becomes far more complex for patients not meeting brain death criteria. Cases involving such situations have involved much legal attention and effort. The issue is further complicated by whether the patient was medically competent or incompetent prior to receiving the life-sustaining support.

States have defined situations in which life-sustaining measures can be withdrawn in various ways. Some states have legislative laws clarifying the procedures to follow; in other states, case law applies. For example, in the state of Washington, for previously competent patients who have not executed a physician's directive or a durable power of attorney, a ventilator may be discontinued if there is unanimous concurrence by the attending physician and two disinterested physicians (determining that the patient's condition is incurable and that there is no reasonable medical probability of the patient's returning to a human state), and the immediate family agrees with the desirability of discontinuing life-sustaining treatment. It is believed that the immediate family is in the best position to address the question of whether the patient, if competent, would have chosen discontinuation of life support.

The question of discontinuation of artificial feeding has not been adequately resolved through either case law or legislative law in most states.

For patients who have been incompetent since birth, a guardian must be appointed who, along with the physician and two disinterested physicians, must be in unanimous agreement that the incompetent patient's best interests are served by termination of life-sustaining treatment.

REFERENCES

1. Guidelines for the determination of brain death: report of the medical consultants on the diagnosis of brain death to the President's Commission for the Study of Ethical Problems in Medicine and Biomedical and Behavioral Research. Neurology 32:395, 1982.

2. A definition of irreversible coma. Report of the Ad Hoc Committee of the Harvard Medical School to examine the definition of brain death. JAMA *205*:337, 1968.
3. Bass E: Cardiopulmonary arrest: pathophysiology and neurologic complications. Ann Intern Med *103*:920, 1985.
4. Miles SH, Cranford R, Schultz AL: The do-not-resuscitate order in a teaching hospital: considerations and a suggested policy. Ann Intern Med *96*:660, 1982.
5. Lipton HL: Do-not-resuscitate decisions in a community hospital. JAMA *256*:1164, 1986.

18

POST-RESUSCITATION CARE

Once a spontaneous and stable perfusing cardiac rhythm is obtained during a resuscitation, subsequent management becomes crucial in maintaining the successful response and minimizing organ damage in order to optimize the patient's overall post-resuscitation status. The following is a recommended approach to post-resuscitation management.

STEPS IN POST-RESUSCITATION MANAGEMENT

1. Maintain Cardiac Rhythm. Continuous ECG monitoring is essential. A perfusing rhythm should be maintained, usually by continuous IV infusion of antiarrhythmic agents as appropriate. This is especially important in patients who had ventricular fibrillation or ventricular tachycardia during the arrest. Patients with hemodynamically unstable bradycardia should have a temporary transvenous pacemaker inserted as soon as possible.

2. Monitor Blood Pressure. Blood pressure must be monitored frequently and systolic blood pressure maintained above 100 mm Hg to minimize further cerebral impairment. Inotropic agents, such as dopamine, should be administered to hypotensive patients until hemodynamic monitoring with a pulmonary artery flow–directed catheter is established, and treatment can be guided by cardiac output and pulmonary artery occluded (pulmonary capillary wedge) pressure measurements.

3. Obtain Arterial Blood Gas Measurements. Adequacy of ventilation and acid-base balance can be assessed by arterial blood gas measurements. The presence either of hypoxia uncorrected by supplemental oxygen or of hypercapnia may be an indication for endotracheal intubation. If the patient is already intubated, readjustment of ventilatory parameters or initiation of positive end-expiratory pressure (PEEP) may be necessary.

Persistent acidosis despite adequate perfusion and ventilation may require bicarbonate therapy. The etiology of the acidosis (e.g., sepsis, renal insufficiency, drug toxicity) must be determined and corrected.

4. Obtain Laboratory Tests. Serum electrolytes, glucose, BUN, creatinine, cardiac enzymes, drug levels, and other appropriate chemistries should be obtained.

5. Obtain ECG. A 12-lead ECG should be obtained as soon as possible and compared with previous tracings, if available. Serial ECGs should be followed as indicated until the pattern stabilizes.

6. Obtain Chest X-Ray. Obtain a portable chest x-ray as soon as possible after resuscitation, to determine ET tube placement and presence of pneumothorax, rib fracture, or other sequelae of cardiac arrest or resuscitation.

7. Consider Nasogastric Tube Insertion. Patients with abdominal distention or absent bowel sounds, or who are intubated should have a nasogastric tube inserted to decompress the stomach.

8. Monitor Urine Output. Urine output must be monitored closely to assess adequacy of renal perfusion and renal function. Short term urinary (Foley) catheterization is usually advised, unless the patient is awake and alert and able to cooperate with urine output monitoring.

MANAGEMENT IN THE INTENSIVE CARE UNIT

Following the steps discussed above, the patient should be transferred to an intensive care setting for continued cardiac monitoring and further evaluation. Patients who are hypotensive need emergent hemodynamic monitoring and can be transferred to an intensive care unit immediately after establishment of a stable and perfusing rhythm. However, the steps listed in the preceding section must still be completed concomitantly with placement of pulmonary artery and intra-arterial lines.

In the intensive care setting, an attempt must be made to establish the etiology of the cardiac arrest. All organ systems should be evaluated, to optimize function and to assess for any damage sustained during the cardiac arrest or the resuscitation efforts.

Evaluation of Organ Systems

Pulmonary. Continue to examine the lungs and monitor chest x-rays for development of pneumothorax, aspiration pneumonitis, pulmonary edema, or shock lung (ARDS—adult respiratory distress syndrome). This is especially important in intubated patients on PEEP. Arterial blood gas measurements should be obtained frequently, to assess adequacy of ventilation and acid-base balance. An intra-arterial catheter facilitates blood sampling and blood pressure monitoring.

Cardiovascular. Hemodynamic monitoring is usually warranted in post–cardiac arrest patients and is mandatory in post-arrest hypotensive patients. Central venous pressure measurements alone are inadequate, since right-sided pressures do not reflect left ventricular filling pressures or function in patients with any pulmonary dysfunction. Cardiac output measurements and pulmonary capillary wedge (PCW) pressures are essential for determining optimal preload, afterload, and fluid therapy.

Serial cardiac enzyme measurements and 12-lead ECGs should be obtained to determine possible myocardial damage that either caused the cardiac arrest or resulted from it. An echocardiogram may be needed to detect development of cardiac tamponade, valvular dysfunction, or myocardial dysfunction. Cardiac catheterization may also be indicated.

Renal. Renal function, urinary output, and urinary sediment should be monitored closely to determine fluid status and monitor for development of acute tubular necrosis (ATN) as a result of cardiac arrest. Dosages of nephrotoxic or predominantly renally excreted drugs must be adjusted depending on renal function.

Central Nervous System. See Chapter 12 (Cerebral Resuscitation).

Gastrointestinal. Closely assess for need of nasogastric tube insertion, if not already inserted. Stress ulceration and bowel ischemia are potential problems, especially if peripheral vasoconstricting drugs are used. Prophylactic use of hourly antacids is strongly recommended. H_2-blocking drugs (cimetidine or ranitidine) can also be used, but their potential CNS side effects may complicate management.

After the patient has been stabilized and within 12–24 hours, all invasive catheters placed in the emergent setting without adequate sterile techniques must be removed and replaced as necessary. The patient must be watched closely for signs of infection. Prophylactic antibiotics are not recommended routinely.

19

DOCUMENTATION

Code sheets are used to document what occurred during a resuscitation. Information contained on code sheets serves five purposes:

1. Medical Records: Documentation of medical therapy becomes a permanent part of the patient's chart.

2. Legal Reasons: As part of the medical record, the flow chart can be reviewed or subpoenaed in medicolegal cases.

3. Research: Research studies to improve resuscitation may use code sheet data.

4. Teaching and Training: The code sheet is valuable in reviewing resuscitations and as a teaching tool for medical and nursing staff.

5. Quality Assurance: Were correct policies, procedures, and protocols followed?

The trick to using a code sheet properly is to use it *during* the code and not after the flurry and drama has subsided. As described in Chapter 2, one team member should be responsible for recording information on the code sheet. In most hospitals, preprinted code sheets are available. Ornato and colleagues have proposed an electronic code sheet to facilitate the recording of data (Ornato JP, et al: Ann Emerg Med *10*:138, 1981).

The important elements of each code sheet, which obviously differ in detail from hospital to hospital, are:

1. Means to record the circumstances of the arrest.

2. A grid that relates time to patient's condition (vital signs, ECG), therapy, lab results, and procedures.

3. Termination of resuscitation and outcome.

4. Signatures of responsible physician and nurse.

Figure 19–1 shows the code sheet used in the University of Washington Hospitals.

DATE	TIME OF ARREST	PATIENT DIAGNOSIS AND SERVICE	PATIENT INTUBATED AT (TIME)
HOW WAS ARREST RECOGNIZED? (ASYTOLE V TACH, ETC.)			COMPLICATIONS

VENTILATION INITIATED AT (TIME)	MOUTH TO MOUTH ☐ YES ☐ NO	ANESTHESIA BAG AND MASK ☐ YES ☐ NO	PATIENT INTUBATED PRIOR TO ARREST ☐ YES ☐ NO	ESTIMATED PERIOD OF APNEA
BY WHOM			EXTERNAL CARDIAC MASSAGE INITIATED AT (TIME)	PRECORDIAL THUMP ☐ YES ☐ NO

TIME	VITAL SIGNS	ATROPINE	BICARB	LIDOCAINE	CALCIUM	EPINEPH.	MS	VALIUM			IV DRIPS	DEFRIBRILLATION			COMMENTS (LAB RESULTS, LOC, PUPILS, ETC.)
												PRE-SHOCK RHYTHM	WATT-SEC	RESULTING RHYTHM	

COMMENTS: (PACEMAKER, IABP, INTERNAL MASSAGE ETC.)	SIGNATURE—R.N.
PRESUMED CAUSE / NATURE OF ARREST	
TERMINATION OF CPR (TIME / RATIONALE / RESULTS)	
FAMILY NOTIFIED	SIGNATURE—PHYSICIAN IN CHARGE

UNIVERSITY OF WASHINGTON HOSPITALS
HARBORVIEW MEDICAL CENTER
UNIVERSITY HOSPITAL
SEATTLE, WASHINGTON

CARDIO PULMONARY ARREST RECORD
CODE 199

ORIGINAL—MED RECORD
DUPLICATE—DEPT. COPY

UH 0665 SEP 79

1-9-3260

Figure 19–1

APPENDICES

APPENDIX I: TABLE OF ACLS DRUGS

Drug	Dosages	Mode of Action	Clinical Use in Emergency Care	Notes
Antiarrhythmics Lidocaine	a. For cardiac arrest: bolus of 1 mg/kg IV, then 0.5 mg/kg every 5–10 min, up to 3 mg/kg b. For noncardiac arrest: bolus of 1 mg/kg IV, then continuous infusion of 2–4 mg/min with infusion pump NOTE: Many recommend a repeat 0.5 mg/kg bolus at 5–10 min for all patients c. Reduce bolus by half in CHF, severe liver disease, shock, age over 70 d. Can also be given via endotracheal tube e. For 4 mg/ml solution, add 1 g to 250 ml D5W	Ventricular antiarrhythmic — decreases automaticity by slowing rate of phase 4 depolarization	a. Control of ventricular premature beats, VT, and VF b. Prophylactic use in acute MI	a. *Contraindications:* idioventricular rhythm, escape mechanism ventricular beats b. *Toxicity:* CNS effects (slurred speech, altered mentation, muscle twitching, seizures); may also produce double vision, numbness, nausea, hypotension

Drug	Dosage	Action	Uses	Nursing considerations
Procainamide hydrochloride (Pronestyl)	a. 100 mg IV every 5 min at rate of 20 mg/min to maximum of 1 g b. Maintenance infusion 1–4 mg/min c. Reduce dosage in renal failure d. For 2 mg/ml solution, add 500 mg to 250 ml D5W	Ventricular antiarrhythmic	a. Recurrent PVCs, VT, and VF refractory to other antiarrhythmics b. Interchangeable with quinidine—not as effective with supraventricular arrhythmias	a. Stop giving drug if QRS complex 50% wider than original or hypotension occurs b. Monitor BP continuously for hypotension, have a vasopressor readily available c. Dilute before giving IV push
Bretylium tosylate (Bretylol)	a. VF or pulseless VT: 5 mg/kg IV bolus, electrical defibrillation. If VF persists, give up to 10 mg/kg and repeat every 15–30 mins, to maximum total dose of 30 mg/kg. Defibrillate after each bolus b. For refractory or recurrent VT: 5–10 mg/kg diluted to 50 ml with D5W, given over 8–10 min, followed by 1–2 mg/min infusion c. For 2 mg/ml solution add 500 mg to 250 ml D5W	a. Ventricular antiarrhythmic b. Postganglionic adrenergic blocker c. Increases VF threshold, action potential duration, and effective refractory period without changing heart rate d. Initial release of catecholamines followed by chemical sympathectomy state	a. Refractory or recurrent VF or unstable VT resistant to lidocaine b. Stable VT resistant to lidocaine and procainamide	a. Monitor BP b. Postural hypotension common c. Onset of anti-VT action may be delayed by 20 min to 2 hours—drug works faster in VF d. May aggravate digoxin toxicity

Table continued on following page

APPENDIX I: TABLE OF ACLS DRUGS *Continued*

Drug	Dosages	Mode of Action	Clinical Use in Emergency Care	Notes
Atropine	a. *For bradycardia:* 0.5 mg IV every 5 min until desired heart rate achieved or a maximum of 2 mg given b. *For asystole:* 1.0 mg bolus IV; repeat in 5 min if needed NOTE: a minimum dose of 0.5 mg *must* be given, as smaller doses *slow* the heart rate c. Can be given intratracheally	a. Parasympathetic blocker—blocks vagal action on SA and AV nodes and increases heart rate	a. Treatment of significant sinus bradycardia with any of the following: 1. Hypotension 2. Frequent ectopic beats 3. Reduced cardiac output 4. Chest pain May be useful in: a. AV block at nodal level b. Ventricular asystole	a. May increase myocardial oxygen demand—use cautiously in acute MI b. May cause VT, VF c. Contraindicated in patients with glaucoma or urinary retention d. Long half-life may cause persisting tachycardia
Verapamil (Isoptin, Calan)	5 mg IV bolus, then 10 mg in 15–30 min if PSVT persists	a. Ca^{++} channel blocker b. Slows conduction and prolongs refractoriness in the AV node	a. Paroxysmal supraventricular tachycardia (PSVT) with nodal conduction. Slows ventricular response in atrial flutter and fibrillation	a. Do not use in Wolff-Parkinson-White syndrome with delta wave or Lown-Ganong-Levine (LGL) with wide QRS b. May have drop in BP and heart rate, and prolonged AV conduction c. May have drop in cardiac output d. Caution in sick sinus syndrome, AV block, and CHF

Drug	Dosage	Action	Use	Nursing implications
				e. Concomitant use of IV Inderal is contraindicated f. Adverse effects may be reversed with CaCl, 0.5–1.0 g IV
Propranolol hydrochloride (Inderal)	1–3 mg IV given slowly every 5 min to total of 0.1 mg/kg	a. β-adrenergic receptor blocking agent b. Direct myocardial depressant c. Slows heart rate and conduction	a. Control of hemodynamically significant atrial tachydysrhythmias b. May be effective in ventricular arrythmias caused by digoxin toxicity c. Use cautiously in patients with acute MI	a. Use extreme caution with patients dependent on β-adrenergic receptor support, especially those with bronchospasm, depressed cardiac function, or 2nd or 3rd degree AVB b. Monitor BP for hypotension c. Observe for bradycardia, heart failure, and hypoglycemia
Adrenergic Agonists Isoproterenol hydrochloride (Isuprel)	a. Infusion rate 2–20 mcg/min titrated to response of rate and rhythm b. For 2 mcg/ml solution, add 1 mg to 500 ml D5W c. For 4 mcg/ml solution, add 1 mg to 250 ml D5W	a. Pure β-adrenergic receptor stimulator b. Increased rate and strength of contractions result in increased myocardial oxygen demand	a. Temporary treatment of hemodynamically significant bradycardia resistant to atropine until pacemaker is inserted	a. Can cause ventricular irritability b. Watch for hypotension due to peripheral vasodilating action, especially if patient is hypovolemic c. In digitalis toxicity, tachydysrhythmia made worse

Table continued on following page

APPENDIX I: TABLE OF ACLS DRUGS *Continued*

Drug	Dosages	Mode of Action	Clinical Use in Emergency Care	Notes
Adrenergic Stimulating Agents				
Epinephrine (Adrenalin)	a. For cardiac arrest: 5–10 ml (0.5–1.0 mg) of 1:10,000 solution IV every 5 min b. Can also be given via endotracheal tube	α- and β-adrenergic stimulation: 1. Peripheral vasoconstriction 2. + inotropic on heart 3. chronotropic on heart	a. For ventricular fibrillation b. To stimulate contraction of heart in asystole c. To increase force of heart contraction in EMD	Short duration of action (5 min)
Norepinephrine (Levophed)	a. 8 mcg/min continuous IV infusion; titrate to BP response b. For 16 mcg/ml solution, add 4 mg to 250 ml D5W c. Use infusion pump	Potent stimulating agent	Severe hypotension or cardiogenic shock not due to hypovolemia	a. Increases myocardial oxygen requirements and may increase area of ischemia and infarction b. Assess volume status first c. Phentolamine (Regitine), 5–10 mg in 10–15 cc saline SC and in same line reverses Levophed extravasation d. Need intra-arterial monitoring e. Contraindicated in patients using MAO inhibitors

Drug	Dosage/Administration	Action	Indications	Considerations
Dopamine hydrochloride (Intropin)	a. 2–20 mcg/kg/min continuous IV infusion b. For 800 mcg/ml solution, add 200 mg to 250 ml D5W c. Use infusion pump	a. α- and β-adrenergic stimulation, and dopamine receptor stimulation b. At 2–10 mcg/kg/min, primarily dopaminergic. At 10–20 mcg/kg/min, α- and β-adrenergic stimulation become active c. At >20 mcg/kg/min, α-adrenergic stimulation reverses effect on dopamine receptors and results in decrease in mesenteric and renal blood flow	Cardiogenic shock and hemodynamically significant hypotension	a. If tachydysrhythmias develop, reduce flow rate b. At very low doses, stimulation of dopamine receptors yields increased renal and mesenteric blood flow c. Hemodynamic monitoring recommended d. Do not give in IV line used for sodium bicarbonate
Dobutamine hydrochloride (Dobutrex)	a. 2.5–10 mcg/kg/min continuous IV infusion b. For 500 mcg/ml solution, add 250 mg to 500 ml D5W c. Use infusion pump	Direct—adrenergic receptor stimulating agent	Short-term use in cardiogenic shock (refractory pump failure)	a. No direct peripheral vasoconstriction, so any increase in BP results from an increase in contractility b. Synergistic with nitroprusside c. Hemodynamic monitoring recommended d. May increase ventricular rate in inadequately treated atrial fibrillation e. Contraindicated in patients with hypertrophic obstructive cardiomyopathy

Table continued on following page

219

APPENDIX I: TABLE OF ACLS DRUGS *Continued*

Drug	Dosages	Mode of Action	Clinical Use in Emergency Care	Notes
Vasodilating Agents				
Intravenous nitroglycerin (Tridil or Nitrobid IV)	a. 10 mcg/min continuous IV infusion, increasing by 5 mcg every 3–5 min b. Follow manufacturer's instructions for preparation of solution c. Use infusion pump	a. Relaxation of vascular smooth muscle b. Venous effect dominant	a. Unstable angina b. Coronary vasospasm (Prinzmetal's angina) c. CHF	a. Drug migrates into plastics. Use glass or McGaw Accumed containers with special tubing and titrate dose by patient response b. Hemodynamic monitoring necessary in patients with CHF
Sodium nitroprusside (Nipride)	a. 0.5–10 mcg/kg/min continuous IV infusion starting with low dose and titrating to desired effect b. For 200 mcg/ml solution, add 50 mg to 250 ml D5W c. Use infusion pump	Direct peripheral vasodilator	a. Hypertension in MI or dissecting aortic aneurysm b. Decrease workload and myocardial oxygen demands in pump failure	a. Intra-arterial monitoring for hypertension b. Hemodynamic monitoring for CHF c. Decomposes on exposure to light; wrap container and tubing with aluminum foil d. Monitor for metabolic acidosis in cyanide poisoning e. Monitor thiocyanate levels, especially in renal insufficiency

Drug	Dose	Action	Indications	Nursing Considerations
Nifedipine (Procardia)	a. For angina: 10 mg PO, increase by 10 mg increments to total of 30 mg over 4–6 h. Maintenance dose, 10–30 mg 3–4 times/day b. For hypertension: 10 mg sublingually; may repeat in 30–60 min	a. Blocks Ca^{++} influx into cell during repolarization b. Produces coronary and peripheral vasodilation	a. Relaxation and prevention of coronary artery spasm b. Some use in acute treatment of hypertension	a. Monitor BP b. Does not prolong AV conduction or slow sinus rate c. May increase serum digoxin level d. May cause peripheral edema
Diuretics Furosemide (Lasix) Ethacrynic acid (Edecrin)	20–40 mg; repeat at higher dose if no effect after 15 min	a. Inhibit sodium reabsorption in kidney b. Some direct vasodilating effect	a. Pulmonary edema b. Cerebral edema after cardiac arrest	a. Must have renal blood flow b. Patients taking oral medication need larger doses
Miscellaneous Digoxin	0.25–0.50 mg IV bolus followed by 0.25 mg IV every 2 h until desired heart rate achieved	a. Vagomimetic action at AV node b. + inotropic effect	Hemodynamically stable atrial fibrillation or atrial flutter	a. Caution in hypokalemia. b. Narrow therapeutic range—monitor serum level c. Toxicity—arrhythmias, especially PVCs, junctional escape rhythms, PAT with block, AV block; GI symptoms d. Decrease dose in renal insufficiency

Table continued on following page

APPENDIX I: TABLE OF ACLS DRUGS *Continued*

Drug	Dosages	Mode of Action	Clinical Use in Emergency Care	Notes
Morphine sulfate	2–5 mg IV every 5–30 min, titrated to desired effect	a. Analgesic b. Vasodilation c. Sedation	a. Treatment of ischemic cardiac pain b. Treatment of pulmonary edema	a. Monitor for respiratory depression and hypotension b. May worsen bradycardia
Calcium chloride	2–5 ml of a 10% solution	Replenishes calcium	Antidote to calcium channel block toxicity and hypocalcemia	a. May precipitate digoxin toxicity b. Precipitates in sodium bicarbonate c. May be detrimental to resuscitation efforts

Drug	Dosage	Action	Indication	Precautions
Sodium bicarbonate	a. 1.0 mEq/kg IV initial dose b. 0.5 mEq/kg IV every 10 min or dose based on ABG results	Direct chemical reversal of acidosis	a. Correct metabolic acidosis from anaerobic metabolism in cardiac arrest b. To obtain optimum pH for defibrillation	a. Need arterial pH to accurately determine dosage b. Excessive dosage produces alkalosis, and ventricular fibrillation may not convert; also, alkalosis impairs release of oxygen from hemoglobin c. Do not mix with other medications d. Should not be used in first 10 min of resuscitation
Amrinone (Inocor)	a. Initial: 0.75 mg/kg bolus slowly over 2–3 min b. Maintenance infusion: 5–10 mcg/kg/min c. For 1 mg/ml solution, add 100 mg (20 ml) to 100 ml NS or ½ NS	Inotropic and vasodilator action	CHF refractory to usual therapy	a. Requires hemodynamic monitoring b. May cause thrombocytopenia c. May increase risk of arrhythmias in CHF d. Do not dilute with dextrose solutions, may inject into running dextrose infusions

APPENDIX II: POCKET SUMMARY OF ACLS DRUGS

This summary drug page can be cut out and used as a pocket guide.

ADVANCED CARDIAC LIFE SUPPORT: DRUGS & DOSAGES

Drug	Indications	Dosage (Adults)
Atropine	Symptomatic bradyarrhythmia or heart block, asystole (1.0 mg IV)	0.5 mg IV every 5 min up to 2 mg
Bicarbonate	Consider for persistent cardiac arrest and/or return of perfusing rhythm	1 mEq/kg IV, then 0.5 mEq/kg every 10 min
Bretylium (Bretylol)	VF or VT not responsive to lidocaine	5 mg/kg IV push. May repeat in 15 min intervals with 10 mg/kg IV (Max of 30 mg/kg)
Calcium Chloride	Not indicated in cardiac arrest	
Digoxin (Lanoxin)	Rapid atrial fib	0.5–1.0 mg IV. May repeat 0.25 mg every 2 hr until effect
Dobutamine (Dobutrex)	Short term inotropic support	2.5–10 mcg/kg/min (250 mg in 500 ml D5W = 500 mcg/ml)
Dopamine (Intropin)	Cardiogenic shock	2–50 mcg/kg/min start at low dose 2–5 mcg/kg/min (200 mg in 250 ml D5W = 800 mcg/ml)
Epinephrine	Asystole, EM dissociation, VF not responding to shocks	0.5–1 mg (10 ml, 1:10,000) IV (or endotracheally or IC). May repeat every 5 min

Table continued on following page

ADVANCED CARDIAC LIFE SUPPORT: DRUGS
& DOSAGES Continued

Drug	Indications	Dosage (Adults)
Isoproterenol (Isuprel)	Symptomatic bradycardia or heart block not responsive to atropine Not indicated in cardiac arrest	2–20 mcg/min (1 mg in 250 ml D5W = 4 mcg/ml) titrated to heart rate
Lidocaine	VF, VT, PVC's	1.0 mg/kg IV push; may repeat every 10 min with 0.5 mg/kg up to 3 mg/kg. Follow with 2–4 mg/min IV drip (1 g in 250 ml D5W = 4 mg/ml)
Nitroglycerine	Unstable angina, CHF	0.4 mg SL every 5 min up to 3 tab 5 mcg/min IV, increasing by 5 mcg/min every 3–5 min up to 500 mcg/min (8 mg in 250 ml D5W = approx 30 mcg/ml; use glass container)
Nitroprusside (Nipride)	Hypertensive crisis, dissecting aortic aneurysm	0.5–15 mcg/kg/min (50 mg in 250 ml D5W = 200 mcg/ml)
Norepinephrine Levarterenol (Levophed)	Cardiogenic shock	8–32 mcg/min start at low dose (4 mg in 250 ml D5W = 16 mcg/ml)
Procainamide (Pronestyl)	VF or VT not responsive to lidocaine or bretylium	100 mg over 5 min IV up to loading dose of 1 g followed by 1–4 mg/min IV drip (500 mg in 250 ml D5W = 2 mg/ml)
Propranolol (Inderal)	VF or VT not responsive to lidocaine, bretylium, or procainamide	1 mg/min diluted in 10 ml D5W IV up to 5 mg
Verapamil	PSVT, temporary control of fast atrial flutter or atrial fib	5–10 mg IV over 1 min; may repeat dose in 15–30 min

APPENDIX III: ABBREVIATED ACLS PROTOCOLS

This appendix contains simplified ACLS protocols as well as mnemonics to assist in remembering the sequence of each protocol.

VENTRICULAR FIBRILLATION (VF)

Shock 200 joules
↓
Shock 200–300 joules
↓
Shock up to 360 joules
↓
Epinephrine 0.5–1.0 mg IV
↓
Shock up to 360 joules
↓
Lidocaine 1 mg/kg IV
↓
Shock up to 360 joules
↓
Bretylium 5 mg/kg IV
↓
Shock up to 360 joules

Mnemonic:

Shock, Shock, Shock, Everybody Shock
Little Shock, Big Shock

VENTRICULAR TACHYCARDIA (VT)

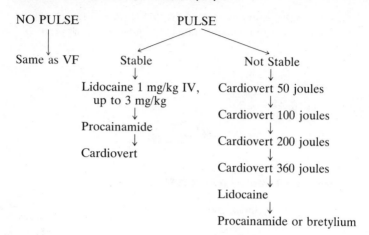

NO PULSE   PULSE

Same as VF   Stable   Not Stable

Stable:
- Lidocaine 1 mg/kg IV, up to 3 mg/kg
- Procainamide
- Cardiovert

Not Stable:
- Cardiovert 50 joules
- Cardiovert 100 joules
- Cardiovert 200 joules
- Cardiovert 360 joules
- Lidocaine
- Procainamide or bretylium

Mnemonic:

> Pulse and awake
> Drugs they must take
>
> Pulse and a nap
> Zap, zap, zap, zap
>
> When shocks can't win
> Let pharmacy begin

ASYSTOLE*

Pacer (as soon as possible)
↓
Epinephrine 0.5–1.0 mg IV
↓
Atropine 1.0 mg IV

Mnemonic:

> Popeye eats asparagus
> Please eat apples

---

*The American Heart Association recommends that pacing be considered after epinephrine and atropine.

ELECTROMECHANICAL DISSOCIATION (EMD)

Epinephrine 0.5–1.0 mg IV
↓
Consider differential
(hypovolemia, tamponade, tension
pneumothorax, embolism, acidosis,
hypoxia)

Mnemonic:

EMD (Epi, memorize differential)

BRADYCARDIA

STABLE   UNSTABLE
↓   ↓
Observe   Atropine 0.5 mg IV up to 2 mg
                              ↓
               External pacemaker (or isoproterenol)
                              ↓
               Transvenous pacemaker

Mnemonic:

First atropine
Then a pace machine

PAROXYSMAL SUPRAVENTRICULAR TACHYCARDIA (PSVT)

UNSTABLE   STABLE
↓   ↓
Cardiovert 75–100 joules   Vagal maneuvers
↓   ↓
Cardiovert 200 joules   Verapamil, 5 mg IV
↓   ↓
Cardiovert 360 joules   Verapamil, 10 mg IV
↓   ↓
Verapamil   Cardioversion, digoxin,
                                beta blockers, pacing

Mnemonic:

If there's time, verapamil
If not, an electric pill

INDEX

Note: Page numbers in *italics* refer to illustrations; page numbers followed by t refer to tables.

ABCs, in basic CPR, 32–38, 35t.
See also *Airway; Breathing; Circulation.*
in pediatric patients, 167–168
Abdominal thrusts, in airway obstruction, 41
Aberrant conduction, vs. premature ventricular contractions, 139t
ABGs. See *Arterial blood gases.*
Acid-base abnormalities, in cardiac arrest, clinical recommendations for, 148
Acid-base balance, 142–148
arterial-venous CO_2 gap and, 142–144
three golden rules of, 144t
application of, 146t
ventilation in, importance of, 142
Acidosis, cerebrospinal fluid, 147
correction of, in cerebral resuscitation, 154
in cardiac arrest, bicarbonate therapy for, controversy regarding, 145–147
in near-drowning, 192
in refractory ventricular fibrillation, 119
ACLS (advanced cardiac life support), drugs used in, 214t–223t. See also names of specific drugs, e.g., *Lidocaine.*
pocket summary of, 225–226
legal considerations in, 201–206
Adrenalin. See *Epinephrine.*
Adrenergic agonists (adrenergic stimulating agents), in ACLS, 217t–219t
in resuscitation, 106–108
Adults, cardiac causes of sudden death in, 8t
Advanced cardiac life support. See *ACLS.*

Advanced life support. See *ALS.*
AED (automatic external defibrillator), 82–83
determination of candidates for, 84, *84*
emergency personnel and, 83–84
Age, as survival factor in cardiac arrest, 11
AID (automatic implantable defibrillator), 83
determination of candidates for, 84, *84*
Airway, establishment of, in infants and children, 167
in basic CPR, initial assessment of, 32
management of, 39–44. See also *Airway management.*
opening of, 33–34
physical maneuvers for, 34
obstruction of, acute, pediatric respiratory arrest due to, 163
CPR measures in, 40–42
Airway control, in advanced life support, 52–55
in basic life support, 47–48
vs. ventilation, 47
Airway management, 45–60. See also *Airway control* and *Ventilation.*
core skills of, for basic and advanced life support personnel, 46t
in basic CPR, 39–44
AHA Standards change in, 42–43
in pediatric patients, 167
in secondary cardiac arrest, 40
with devices, personnel approach in, 46–47, 46t
without devices, 45, 46t
Alkalosis, in refractory ventricular fibrillation, 119

ALS (advanced life support), airway control in, 52–55
  airway management in, 46–47, 46t
  devices used in, 51–57
  cricothyrotomy in, 56–57
  endotracheal intubation in, 53–55
  in near-drowning, 194
  in pediatric patients, 168–173
  transtracheal catheter insufflation in, 55
  ventilation in, 55–57
Amrinone, 113
  in ACLS, 223t
Anectine, in pediatric endotracheal intubation, 173
Antiarrhythmics, in ACLS, 214t–217t
  in resuscitation, 103–105, 214t–217t
Anticipation phase (phase I), in code organization, 26–27, 27
Arrest, cardiac. See Cardiac arrest.
  circulatory, 15, 17
  near, features of, 17
  respiratory, 17, 163–165
Arrest time, and neurologic outcome, 149, 152
Arrhythmias, 114–141. See also names of specific types, e.g., Ventricular fibrillation (VF).
  management of, guidelines and protocols for, 114–115
Arterial blood gases (ABGs), evaluation of, in cardiac arrest, 144
  measurement of, in mechanical ventilation, 58
  post-resuscitation, 208
Artifact, excessive, in defibrillation, causes of, 79–80
Aspiration, of foreign body, pediatric respiratory arrest due to, 163–164
Asynchronous mode, in defibrillation, 77
Asystole, 123–125
  diagnosis of, 123–124
  post-defibrillation, transcutaneous pacemaker for, 95, 95t
  therapy for, 124–125, 125
  transcutaneous pacemaker for, 95, 95t

Atrial fibrillation, 131–134
  causes of, 132t
  diagnosis of, 131–132, 132t
  ECG in, 132
  therapy for, 132–134
    elective cardioversion in, 133–134
    emergency cardioversion in, 133
Atrial flutter, 130–131
  causes of, 130t
  diagnosis of, 130, 130t
  ECG in, 130
  therapy for, 130–131
Atrioventricular (AV) block, first-degree, causes of, 134t
    diagnosis of, 134t
    ECG in, 135
    therapy for, 136, 137
  second-degree, Mobitz Type I (Wenckebach), causes of, 135t
    diagnosis of, 135t
    ECG in, 135
    therapy for, 136, 137
  Mobitz Type II, causes of, 136t
    diagnosis of, 136t
    ECG in, 136
    therapy for, 136, 137
  third-degree (complete heart block), causes of, 136t
    diagnosis of, 136t
    ECG in, 136
    therapy for, 136, 137
Atropine, 104–105
  in ACLS, 216t, 225
  in pediatric patients, 175t
Authorization form, physician's, to withhold or limit therapeutic measures, 203
AV block, 134–137. See also Atrioventricular (AV) block.

Bag-valve-mask unit, with oxygen, 49–50
  FATS (face and thigh squeeze) technique for, 50t
Barbiturates, in cerebral resuscitation, 160
Basic life support. See BLS.

Bicarbonate, 112–113
  in ACLS, 223t, 225
  in cardiac arrest, controversy regarding, 145–148
  in pediatric patients, 175t
Block, atrioventricular, 134–137. See also *Atrioventricular (AV) block.*
Blood chemistries, normalization of, in cerebral resuscitation, 157
Blood gases, arterial. See *Arterial blood gases (ABGs).*
Blood glucose levels, after cardiac arrest, and probability of awakening, 20t
Blood pressure, monitoring of, post-resuscitation, 208
BLS (basic life support), airway control in, 47–48
  airway management in, 45–46, 46t
  devices used in, 47–51
  in pediatric patients, 166–168
  oxygen supplementation in, 50–51
  controversial devices for, 51
  ventilation in, 48–50
Bradyasystolic cardiac arrest, transcutaneous pacing for, 96, 97t, *98*
Bradycardia, 134–137
  ACLS protocol for, 229
  asymptomatic, transcutaneous pacemaker for, 94–95, 95t
  junctional, therapy for, 136
  sinus, causes of, 134t
    diagnosis of, 134, 134t
    ECG in, *134*
    therapy for, 136
  symptomatic, transcutaneous pacemaker for, 94, 95t
Brain. See also *Cerebral resuscitation.*
  damage to, in cardiac arrest, 149
  ischemia of, global, 149
  pathophysiology of, 150–153
Breathing, assessment of, 34
  basic CPR measures for, 34–36
    AHA Standards change in, 36
  in pediatric patients, 167
Bretylium, 104
  in ACLS, 215t, 225
  in pediatric patients, 175t

Buffers, in cardiac arrest, 145–147. See also *Bicarbonate.*
Bypass, cardiopulmonary, in cerebral resuscitation, 161
Bystander(s), as survival factor in cardiac arrest, 11
  CPR initiation by, 12
  vs. delayed CPR, 13t

Calan. See *Verapamil.*
Calcium chloride, 112
  in ACLS, 222t, 225
  in pediatric patients, 175t
Calcium-entry blocking drugs, in cerebral resuscitation, 160
Cannula, nasal, 50
Cannulation, of femoral vein, 65–67, *66*
  of internal jugular vein, 61–63, *63*
  of subclavian vein, 63–65, *64*
Cardiac arrest, 17
  acid-base balance in, 142–148. See also *Acid-base balance.*
    abnormalities of, clinical recommendations for, 148
  acidosis in, bicarbonate therapy for, controversy regarding, 145–147
  anticipation of, 18–19
  arterial-venous CO_2 gap in, 142–144, *143*
  bradyasystolic, transcutaneous pacing for, 96, 97t, *98*
  cerebral resuscitation in, 149–162. See also *Cerebral resuscitation.*
  code organization in, 26–31. See also *Code organization.*
  coma in, probability of awakening from, 19, 20t
  definition of, 7, 15
  due to heart disease, outcomes following, 23t
  duration of, and neurologic outcome, 149, 152
  features of, 17
  global brain ischemia due to, 149
  hypothermia-induced, treatment of, 199

Cardiac arrest *(Continued)*
  in infants and children. See *Pediatric cardiac arrest.*
  in-hospital, survival factors in, 14–15
    survival rates in, 16t
  long-term survival after, 19, 21t
  morbidity after, measures of, 23
    statistics on, 22t
  neurologic outcome after, 19, 149, 152
  out-of-hospital, survival from, 10–11
    fate factors in, 11–12
    program factors in, 12–14, 13t
  outcomes following, 19–23
  pediatric. See *Pediatric cardiac arrest.*
  positioning of patient in, for basic CPR, 33
  prevention of, 18–19
  resuscitation in. See *CPR.*
  secondary, airway management in, 40
  seizures in, prevention of, 156–157
    treatment of, 156–157
  sudden. See also *Cardiac death, sudden.*
    definition of, 15
    outcome of, program factors in, 12–14, 13t
    pathophysiology of, 9–10
    patient in, 7–25
    survival rates in. See *Survival rates, in sudden cardiac arrest.*
  traumatic, 183–191. See also *Traumatic cardiac arrest.*
  types of, 15–17
  witnessed, survival rate in, 11
Cardiac death, sudden. See also *Cardiac arrest, sudden.*
  definition of, 7, 15
  due to infarct, 10t
  due to ischemia, 10t
  etiology of, 8, 8t
  out-of-hospital, epidemiology of, 7
  rhythm associated with, 7
  risk factors in, 8–9
  syndromes of, 10t

Cardiac massage, open-chest, 43–44
Cardiac pacing, emergency, 90–102. See also *Pacemakers* and *Pacing, cardiac.*
Cardiac rhythm(s). See also names of specific rhythms, e.g., *Ventricular fibrillation.*
  as survival factor in sudden cardiac arrest, 11–12
    in paramedic-treated cases, 12t
  in sudden cardiac death, 7
  post-resuscitation maintenance of, 208
Cardiogenic shock, pediatric cardiac arrest due to, 166
Cardiopulmonary bypass, in cerebral resuscitation, 161
Cardiopulmonary resuscitation. See *CPR.*
Cardiovascular monitoring, in cerebral resuscitation, 158
Cardiovascular system, evaluation of, post-resuscitation, 209–210
Cardioversion, cough, 80–81
  for atrial fibrillation, 133–134
  for paroxysmal supraventricular tachycardia, 129
  in pediatric patients, 171–173
Catecholamine stimulation, excessive, in refractory ventricular fibrillation, 120
Catheter(s), transtracheal, insufflation of, 55
Catheterization, intravenous. See *Cannulation.*
Central nervous system. See *CNS.*
Central venous lines, 61–70. See also *Cannulation.*
Cerebral resuscitation, 149–162
  acidosis in, correction of, 154
  barbiturates in, 160
  blood chemistries in, 157
  brain-specific therapies in, experimental, 159–161
  calcium-entry blocking drugs in, 160
  cardiopulmonary bypass in, 161
  cardiovascular monitoring in, 158
  CNS evaluation in, 158–159
  corticosteroids in, 157
  dimethyl sulfoxide in, 161

Cerebral resuscitation *(Continued)*
 fluid balance in, 158
 free iron chelators in, 160–161
 free radical scavengers in, 160
 hematocrit in, 157
 hyperventilation in, 154–156
 immobilization in, 156
 intracranial pressure monitoring
  in, 158
 naloxone in, 161
 normotension in, maintenance
  of, 154
 normothermia in, 157
 nutritional support in, 158
 osmotherapy in, 158
 oxygenation in, 156
 pathophysiologic principles in,
  150–153
 patient position in, 158
 prostaglandin inhibitors in, 160
 sedation in, 156
 seizures in, prevention and treatment of, 156–157
 standard brain-oriented intensive
  care in, 154–159, 155t
 therapeutic approach to, 153–
  161, 155t
 thromboxane antagonists in, 160
Charge button, on defibrillator, 76
Chest compressions, closed, in
  basic CPR, 37
Chest x-ray, post-resuscitation, 209
Children, cardiac arrest in, 163–
  182. See also *Pediatric cardiac
  arrest.*
Chin lift, 34
Choking, basic CPR measures in,
  41–42
 AHA Standards change in,
  42–43
Circulation, assessment of, pulse
  check in, 36
 closed-chest compressions for, 37
 in basic CPR, 36–38
 support of, in infants and children, 167–168
Circulatory arrest, definition of, 15
 traumatic, definition of, 17
Closed-chest compressions, in basic
  CPR, 37
CNS (central nervous system),
  depression of, pediatric respiratory arrest due to, 164

CNS (central nervous system)
  (Continued)
 evaluation of, Glasgow-Pittsburgh Coma Score in, 159t
 in cerebral resuscitation, 158–
  159
Code organization, 26–31
 phase I (anticipation) in, 26, 26–
  27, *27*
 phase II (entry) in, 28
 phase III (resuscitation) in, 28–
  29
 phase IV (maintenance) in, 30
 phase V (family notification) in,
  30
 phase VI (transfer) in, 31
 phase VII (critique) in, 31
Code sheets, 211, *212*
Coma, probability of awakening
  from, calculation of, 19, 20t
Coma Score, Glasgow-Pittsburgh,
  159t
Compressions, closed-chest, in
  basic CPR, 37
Conduction, aberrant, vs. premature ventricular contractions,
  139t
Continuous positive airway pressure (CPAP), in mechanical
  ventilation, 58
Corticosteroids, in cerebral resuscitation, 157
Cough cardioversion, 80–81
Counting approach, in basic CPR,
  38–39
CPAP (continuous positive airway
  pressure), in mechanical ventilation, 58
CPR (cardiopulmonary resuscitation), basic, 32–44
 ABCs in, 32–38. See also *Airway; Breathing; Circulation.*
 counting approach in, 38–39
 one-person, 32–38, 35t
 positioning of patient in, 33
 positioning of rescuer in, 33
 two-person, 38–39
 ventilation/compression ratio
  in, 38–39
 bystander initiation of, 12
  vs. delayed CPR, and outcome in cardiac arrest, 13t
 complications of, 115

CPR (cardiopulmonary resuscitation) *(Continued)*
  duration of, and neurologic outcome, 149, 152
  history of, 1–6
  in pediatric patients, 166–168
    legal considerations in, 201–204
  legal considerations in, 201–206
  low-flow versus no-flow controversy in, 152–153
  open-chest cardiac massage in, 43–44
  termination of, legal considerations in, 204–205
  ventilation in, importance of, 142
  withholding of, legal considerations in, 204
CPR time, and neurologic outcome, 149, 152
Cricothyrotomy, 56–57
Critical care, legal questions in, 201–206
Critique phase (phase VII), in code organization, 31

Death, sudden cardiac. See *Cardiac death, sudden.*
Defibrillation, 70–85. See also *Defibrillators.*
  common errors in, 79t
  cough cardioversion and, 81
  decreasing resistance in, 71–73
  electrical principles in, 71
  electrode gels in, 72
  electrode metal in, 73
  energy levels recommended for, 74–75
  excessive artifact in, causes of, 79–80
  excessive 60-cycle interference in, 80
  future directions in, 80–84
  history of, 2
  in pediatric patients, 171–173
  intrathoracic volume in, 72
  Kite's apparatus for, 2, *4*
  monitor cable movement in, excessive artifact due to, 80
  paddle diameter in (adult), 72
  paddle pressure in, 72–73

Defibrillation *(Continued)*
  physiology of, 71–74
  poor monitor lead-skin contact in, excessive artifact due to, 79
  precordial thump and, 80–81
  problems in, troubleshooting of, 78–80
  rhythm assessment cycle in, 77
  shocks delivered in, number of, 73
    time period between, 73
  technique of, 77–78
  treatment cycle in, 78
  unsnapped monitor leads in, excessive artifact due to, 79
Defibrillators, 74–77. See also *Defibrillation.*
  asynchronous mode of, 77
  automatic external (AED), 82–83
    determination of candidates for, 84, *84*
    emergency personnel and, 83–84
  automatic implantable (AID), 83
    determination of candidates for, 84, *84*
  charge button on, 76
  discharge buttons on, 76
  electrode metal used in, 73
  energy-select switch on, 76
  lead-select switch on, 76
  operating controls of, 75–77
  power-on switch on, 76
  size of ECG on monitor display of, interpretations of, 77
  synchronization button on, 76–77
  synchronized mode of, 77
  waveforms in, 74
Defibrillatory shocks, for ventricular fibrillation, 115
Diazepam, in pediatric endotracheal intubation, 173
Digoxin, 111–112
  in ACLS, 221t, 225
Dimethyl sulfoxide, in cerebral resuscitation, 161
Discharge buttons, on defibrillator, 76
Diuretics, in ACLS, 221t
  in resuscitation, 111, 221t
DNR (Do Not Resuscitate) orders, 204

Do Not Resuscitate (DNR) orders, 204
Dobutamine, 108
  in ACLS, 219t, 225
  pediatric dosage of, 180t, 181t
Dobutrex. See *Dobutamine*.
Documentation, code sheets for, 211, *212*
Dopamine, 107–108
  in ACLS, 219t, 225
Down-time, and neurologic outcome, 149
Drowning, definition of, 192
  delayed, 192
  incidence of, 192
  near-, 192–195. See also *Near-drowning*.
  secondary, 192
Drugs. See also names of specific agents, e.g., *Atropine*.
  in ACLS, 214t–223t, 225–226
  in resuscitation, 103–113

ECG (electrocardiogram), in atrial fibrillation, *132*
  in atrial flutter, *130*
  in atrioventricular block, *135*, *136*
  in idioventricular rhythm, *127*
  in paroxysmal supraventricular tachycardia, *128*
  in premature ventricular contractions, *138*
  in sinus bradycardia, *134*
  in torsade de pointes, *123*
  in ventricular fibrillation, *117*
  in ventricular flutter, *121*
  post-resuscitation, 208
  size of, on defibrillator monitor display, 77
Edecrin (ethacrynic acid), 111
  in ACLS, 221t
Edema, pulmonary, in near-drowning, 192, 193
Electric current, peak, in defibrillation, 71
Electrical capture, in transcutaneous cardiac pacing, 93–94
Electrical principles, in defibrillation, 71
Electrocardiogram. See *ECG*.

Electrode(s), in transcutaneous cardiac pacing, 93
Electrode gels, in defibrillation, 72
Electrode metal, in defibrillation, 73
Electromechanical dissociation (EMD), 125–126
  ACLS protocol for, 229
  diagnosis of, 125–126
  identification of, 126
  therapy for, 126, *126*
EMD. See *Electromechanical dissociation*.
Emergency cardiac pacing, 90–102. See also *Pacemakers* and *Pacing, cardiac*.
Emergency Medical System (EMS), activation of, 36–37
EMS (Emergency Medical System), activation of, 36–37
Encephalopathy, post-ischemic, 149
Endotracheal intubation, 53–55
  in pediatric patients, 168–170, *169*, *170*
  adjunctive medications for, 173
  tube sizes in, 172t
Energy-select switch, on defibrillator, 76
Entry phase (phase II), in code organization, 28
Epiglottitis, pediatric respiratory arrest due to, 164
Epinephrine, 106–107
  in ACLS, 218t, 225
  in pediatric patients, 175t
Ethacrynic acid, 111
  in ACLS, 221t
Eye movements, spontaneous, after cardiac arrest, and probability of awakening, 20t

Face masks, 48–51
Family notification phase (phase V), in code organization, 30
FATS (face and thigh squeeze) technique, for bag-valve-mask ventilation, 50t
Femoral vein, cannulation of, 65–67, *66*

Fibrillation. See *Atrial fibrillation*; *Ventricular fibrillation.*
Finger-sweep maneuver, in airway obstruction, 41
FIO₂, in mechanical ventilation, 58
Fluid balance, in cerebral resuscitation, 158
Foreign body aspiration, pediatric respiratory arrest due to, 163–164
Free iron chelators, in cerebral resuscitation, 160–161
Free radical scavengers, in cerebral resuscitation, 160
Furosemide, 111
  in ACLS, 221t
  in pediatric patients, 175t

Gastrointestinal system, evaluation of, post-resuscitation, 210
Gel(s), electrode, in defibrillation, 72
Global brain ischemia, in cardiac arrest, 149

Head tilt, 34
Heart. See also *Cardiac* entries.
  disease of, cardiac arrest due to, outcomes following, 23t
Heimlich maneuver, in airway obstruction, 41
Hematocrit, normalization of, in cerebral resuscitation, 157
Hospitalized patients, cardiac arrest in, survival rates in, 16t
Hypertension, treatment of, in cerebral resuscitation, 154
Hyperventilation, in cerebral resuscitation, 154–156
Hypokalemia, in refractory ventricular fibrillation, 120
Hypomagnesemia, in refractory ventricular fibrillation, 120
Hypotension, treatment of, in cerebral resuscitation, 154
Hypothermia, 196–200
  clinical features of, 196–197
  definition of, 196
  etiology of, 196
  J wave in, 197

Hypothermia *(Continued)*
  treatment of, 197–199
    general principles in, 197–198
    in mild to moderate cases, 198
    in severe cases, 199
    prehospital, 198
Hypovolemic shock, pediatric cardiac arrest due to, 166
Hypoxia, in near-drowning, 192
Hypoxia time, and neurologic outcome, 149

ICP (intracranial pressure), monitoring of, in cerebral resuscitation, 158
Idioventricular rhythm, 127
  causes of, 127t
  diagnosis of, 127, 127t
  ECG in, *127*
  therapy for, 127
Immersion syndrome, 192
Immobilization, in cerebral resuscitation, 156
Inderal. See *Propranolol.*
Infants, cardiac arrest in, 163–182. See also *Pediatric cardiac arrest.*
Infarct(s), sudden cardiac death due to, 10t
Injection, intracardiac, 87–89
Injury(ies), to operator in transcutaneous pacing, 99
Inocor, in ACLS, 223t
Inspiratory flow rate, in mechanical ventilation, 58
Inspired oxygen concentration (FIO₂), in mechanical ventilation, 58
Insufflation, transtracheal catheter, 55
Internal jugular vein, cannulation of, 61–63, *63*
Intracardiac injection, 87–89
Intracranial pressure (ICP), monitoring of, in cerebral resuscitation, 158
Intrathoracic volume, in defibrillation, 72
Intravenous (IV) lines, 61–70. See also *Cannulation.*
Intropin. See *Dopamine.*
Intubation. See specific type, e.g., *Endotracheal intubation.*

Ischemia, sudden cardiac death due to, 10t
Isoproterenol, 106
 in ACLS, 217t, 226
 pediatric dosage of, 180t
Isoptin. See *Verapamil.*
Isuprel, in ACLS, 217t, 226
 pediatric dosage of, 180t
IV (intravenous) lines, 61–70. See also *Cannulation.*

J wave, in hypothermia, *197*
Jaw thrust, 34
Jugular vein, internal, cannulation of, 61–63, *63*
Junctional bradycardia, therapy for, 136

Kidney(s), evaluation of, post-resuscitation, 210
Kite's apparatus, for electrical resuscitation, 2, *4*

Laboratory tests, post-resuscitation, 208
Lanoxin (digoxin), in ACLS, 221t, 225
Lasix (furosemide), 111
 in ACLS, 221t
Lead-select switch, on defibrillator, 76
Legal considerations, 201–207
Levophed (norepinephrine), 107
 pediatric dosage of, 180t
Lidocaine, 103
 in ACLS, 214t, 226
 in pediatric patients, 175t
Life-sustaining systems, withdrawal of, legal considerations in, 205–206
Lung(s), disease of, pediatric respiratory arrest due to, 165
 edema of, in near-drowning, 192, 193
 evaluation of, post-resuscitation, 209

Maintenance phase (phase IV), in code organization, 30
Mask(s), bag-valve unit with, 49–50
 FATS (face and thigh squeeze) technique for, 50t
 face, 48–51
 Venturi, 51
MAST (Military or Medical Antishock Trousers), 188–191, *186–191*
Mechanical capture, in transcutaneous cardiac pacing, 93–94
Mechanical ventilation, 57–59. See also *Ventilators.*
Medical Antishock Trousers. See *MAST.*
Medical history of patient, as survival factor in cardiac arrest, 11
Medical record, resuscitation code sheet in, 211
Medicolegal cases, resuscitation code sheet in, 211
Military Antishock Trousers. See *MAST.*
Mobitz Types I and II atrioventricular block. See *Atrioventricular (AV) block, second-degree.*
Morbidity, after cardiac arrest, measures of, 23
 statistics on, 22t
Morphine, 112
 in ACLS, 222t
Motor response, after cardiac arrest, and probability of awakening, 20t

Naloxone, in cerebral resuscitation, 161
Nasal cannula, 50
Nasal trumpet device, 48
Nasogastric intubation, in pediatric patients, 170
 tube sizes for, 172t
 in post-resuscitation care, 209
Nasopharyngeal airway device, 48
Nasotracheal tubes, taping of, in infants and children, *170*
Near arrest, 17–18

Near-drowning, 192–195
  clinical presentation of, 192–193
  incidence of, 192
  prognosis in, 195
  treatment of, emergency department procedures for, 194–195, 194t
    initial (prehospital), 193–194
      advanced life support procedures in, 194
Nebulizer therapy, with mechanical ventilation, 59
Neurologic status, after cardiac arrest, 19, 149, 152
Nifedipine, 110–111
  in ACLS, 221t
Nipride. See *Nitroprusside.*
Nitrobid IV. See *Nitroglycerin, intravenous.*
Nitroglycerin, 108–110
  intravenous, in ACLS, 220t, 226
Nitroprusside, 110
  in ACLS, 220t, 226
  pediatric dosage of, 180t
No-Code documentation policy form, *202–203*
Noninvasive cardiac pacing. See *Pacing, cardiac, transcutaneous.*
Norepinephrine, 107
  in ACLS, 218t, 226
Normotension, maintenance of, in cerebral resuscitation, 154
Normothermia, maintenance of, in cerebral resuscitation, 157–158
Nutritional support, in cerebral resuscitation, 158

One-rescuer basic CPR, 32–38, 35t
Open-chest cardiac massage, 43–44
Organ systems, evaluation of, 209–210
Oropharyngeal airway device, 47–48
Orotracheal tubes, taping of, in pediatric patients, *169*
Osborn wave, in hypothermia, *197*
Osmotherapy, in cerebral resuscitation, 158
Overdrive pacing, by transcutaneous pacemaker, indications for, 95–96, 95t

Oxygen supplementation, in basic life support, 50–51
  controversial devices for, 51
Oxygenation, maintenance of, in cerebral resuscitation, 156

Pacemakers, asynchronous, 91
  comparative features of, 92t
  demand, 91
  synchronous, 91
  transcutaneous, 90–100
    asynchronous mode for, 91
    complications of, 92t, 96–99
    contraindications to, 92t
    device controls with, 93
    disadvantages of, 92t
    electrical capture with, 93–94
    electrodes used with, 93
    features of, 92t
    for asymptomatic bradycardias, 94, 94–95, 95t
    for asystole, 95
    for bradyasystolic cardiac arrest, 96, 97t, *98*
    for post-defibrillation asystole, 95, 95t
    for pulseless idioventricular rhythm, 95, 95t
    for symptomatic bradycardias, 94, 95t
    for ventricular standstill (asystole), 95, 95t
    indications for, 94–96, 95t
    mechanical capture with, 93–94
    overdrive pacing by, 95–96, 95t
    rhythm display with, 93
    synchronized demand mode for, 91
  transthoracic, 101–102
    complications of, 92t
    contraindications to, 92t
    disadvantages of, 92t
    features of, 92t
    insertion of, equipment and supplies for, 101
    procedure for, 101–102
  transvenous, 100–101
    complications of, 92t
    contraindications to, 92t
    disadvantages of, 92t

Pacemakers *(Continued)*
transvenous, features of, 92t
insertion of, 100–101
equipment and supplies for, 100
procedure for, 100–101
Pacing, cardiac, 90
transcutaneous, 90
electrical capture in, 93–94
equipment for, 91–94. See
also *Pacemakers, transcutaneous.*
induction of ventricular fibrillation due to, 97
mechanical capture in, 93–
94
operator injuries from, 99
pain due to, 98
perspectives on, 99–100
single-rescuer sequence for, 96
tissue damage due to, 98–99
uses for, 90
Paddle diameter, adult, in defibrillation, 72
Paddle pressure, in defibrillation, 72–73
Pain, due to transcutaneous pacemakers, 98
Pancuronium chloride, in pediatric
endotracheal intubation, 173
Parasympathetic stimulation, excessive, in refractory ventricular fibrillation, 119–120
Parenchyma of lung, disease of,
pediatric respiratory arrest due
to, 165
Paroxysmal supraventricular tachycardia (PSVT), 127–129
ACLS protocol for, 229
causes of, 128t
diagnosis of, 127, 128t
ECG in, *128*
therapy for, *128*, 128–129
cardioversion in, 129
pharmacologic, 129
physical maneuvers in, 128
Patient, positioning of, for basic
CPR, 33
in cerebral resuscitation, 158
Patient history, as survival factor
in cardiac arrest, 11

Pavulon, in pediatric endotracheal
intubation, 173
Peak electric current, in defibrillation, 71
Pediatric cardiac arrest, advanced
life support in, 168–173
basic life support in, 166–168
cause(s) of, 165–166
acquired heart disease as, 166
congenital heart disease as, 166
shock as, 166
vagal stimulation as, 165
emergency medications in, 175t
infusion of, 180t, 182
rule of 6s for, 181t
intravenous access in, 173–179
respiratory arrest and, 163–165
Pediatric respiratory arrest, causes
of, 163–165
PEEP (positive end-expiratory
pressure), in mechanical ventilation, 58
Pericardiocentesis, 86–87
needle insertion in, *88*
Phases in code organization. See
under *Code organization.*
Physician's authorization form, to
withhold or limit therapeutic
measures, *203*
PIVR (pulseless idioventricular
rhythm), transcutaneous
pacemaker in, 95, 95t
Plastic face mask, 50
Pocket face mask, 48–49
Positioning, patient, for basic
CPR, 33
in cerebral resuscitation, 158
Positive end-expiratory pressure
(PEEP), in mechanical venti-
lation, 58
Post-defibrillation asystole, trans-
cutaneous pacemaker for, 95, 95t
Post-ischemic encephalopathy, 149
Post-resuscitation care, 208–210
Post-resuscitation hypoxia time,
and neurologic outcome, 149
Post-resuscitation syndrome, 149
Power-on switch, on defibrillator, 76

Pre-arrest hypoxia time, and neu-
    rologic outcome, 149
Precordial thump, 80–81
Premature ventricular contractions
    (PVCs), 137–140
  causes of, 138t
  diagnosis of, 137–138, 138t
  ECG in, *138*
  therapy for, *138*, 138–140, 139t,
    140
  vs. aberrantly conducted beats,
    139t
Pressure-cycled ventilators, 57
Procainamide, 103–104
  in ACLS, 215t, 226
Procardia (nifedipine), in ACLS,
    221t
Pronestyl, in ACLS, 215t, 226
Propranolol, 105–106
  in ACLS, 217t, 226
Prostaglandin inhibitors, in cere-
    bral resuscitation, 160
PSVT. See *Paroxysmal supraven-
    tricular tachycardia.*
Pulmonary disease, pediatric respi-
    ratory arrest due to, 165
Pulmonary edema, in near-drown-
    ing, 192, 193
Pulmonary function, evaluation of,
    post-resuscitation, 209
Pulse check, in basic CPR, 36
Pulseless idioventricular rhythm
    (PIVR), transcutaneous
    pacemaker for, 95, 95t
Pupillary light response, after car-
    diac arrest, and probability of
    awakening, 20t
PVCs. See *Premature ventricular
    contractions.*

Reanimation chair, in history of
    resuscitation, 2, *6*
Regitine, pediatric dosage of, 180t
Renal function, evaluation of,
    post-resuscitation, 210
Research, resuscitation code sheets
    in, 211
Respiratory arrest, features of, 17
  pediatric, causes of, 163–165
Resuscitation, cardiopulmonary.
    See *CPR.*
  care following, 208–210

Resuscitation *(Continued)*
  cerebral. See *Cerebral resuscita-
    tion.*
  documentation of, 211, *212*
  drugs used in, 103–113. See also
    names of specific drugs, e.g.,
    Lidocaine.
  history of, 1–6
  milestones in, 5t
  legal considerations in, 201–206
Resuscitation phase (phase III), in
    code organization, 28–29
Resuscitation time, and neurologic
    outcome, 149, 152
Rhythm(s), cardiac. See *Cardiac
    rhythm(s)* and specific types,
    e.g., *Ventricular fibrillation.*
Rhythm assessment cycle, in defi-
    brillation, 77

Secondary drowning, 192
Sedation, in cerebral resuscitation,
    156
Seizures, in cardiac arrest, preven-
    tion of, 156–157
  treatment of, 156–157
Septic shock, pediatric cardiac ar-
    rest due to, 166
Sex, as survival factor in cardiac
    arrest, 11
Shock(s), defibrillatory, for ven-
    tricular fibrillation, 115
Shock-related pediatric cardiac ar-
    rest, 166
Sinus bradycardia. See *Bradycar-
    dia, sinus.*
Sodium bicarbonate. See *Bicarbo-
    nate.*
Subclavian vein, cannulation of,
    63–65, *64*
Succinylcholine chloride, in pediat-
    ric endotracheal intubation,
    173
Survival, long-term, after cardiac
    arrest, 19, 21t
Survival determinants, in out-of-
    hospital cardiac arrest, 10–14
Survival rates, in sudden cardiac
    arrest, age and, 11
  among hospitalized patients,
    16t

Survival rates *(Continued)*
  in sudden cardiac arrest, by-
      stander initiation of CPR
      and, 12
    vs. delayed CPR, 13t
  cardiac rhythm and, 11
  paramedic vs. EMT care and,
      12
  prior medical condition and,
      11
  sex and, 11
  time from collapse to defini-
      tive care and, 12–14
  time from collapse to initiation
      of CPR and, 12
  witnessed collapse and, 11
Switches, defibrillator, use of, 76
Synchronization button, on defi-
    brillator, 76–77
Synchronized mode, in defibrilla-
    tion, 77

Teaching, resuscitation code sheets
    as tool in, 211
Thromboxane antagonists, in cere-
    bral resuscitation, 160
Tidal volume, in mechanical venti-
    lation, 58
Time-cycled ventilators, 57
Tissue damage, due to transcutane-
    ous pacemakers, 98–99
Torsade de pointes, 123
  ECG in, *123*
Training, resuscitation code sheets
    in, 211
Transcutaneous pacemakers, 90–
    100. See also *Pacemakers,
    transcutaneous.*
Transfer phase (phase VI), in code
    organization, 31
Transthoracic pacemakers. See
    Pacemakers, transthoracic.
Transtracheal catheter insufflation,
    55
Transvenous pacemakers. See
    Pacemakers, transvenous.
Traumatic cardiac arrest, 183–191
  emergency thoracotomy in, 183–
      186, *184*
  equipment and supplies for,
      184t
  general considerations in, 183

Traumatic cardiac arrest *(Contin-
    ued)*
  initial therapy in, 183–191
  MAST (Military or Medical An-
      tishock Trousers) in, 188–191,
      186–191
  outcome in, 191
Traumatic circulatory arrest, 17
Treatment cycle, in defibrillation,
    78
Tridil (intravenous nitroglycerin),
    in ACLS, 220t
Tube(s). See specific types, e.g.,
    Orotracheal tubes.
Two-rescuer basic CPR, 38–39

Uniform Determination of Death,
    205
Urine output, monitoring of, in
    post-resuscitation care, 209

Vagal stimulation, pediatric cardiac
    arrest due to, 165
Valium, in pediatric endotracheal
    intubation, 173
Vasodilating agents, in ACLS,
    220t–221t
  in resuscitation, 108–111, 220t–
      221t
Vasogenic shock, pediatric cardiac
    arrest due to, 166
Venous cannulation, 61–67, *63, 64,
    66*
Venous cutdown, 67–69, *68, 69*
Ventilation, in acid-base balance,
    importance of, 142
  in advanced life support, 55–57
  in basic CPR, 35
    AHA Standards change in, 36
  in basic life support, 48–50
  in infants and children, 167
  mechanical impairment of, pedi-
      atric respiratory arrest due to,
      165
  mechanical support of, 57–59.
      See also *Ventilators.*
  restriction of, pediatric cardiac
      arrest due to, 165
  vs. airway control, 47
Ventilation/compression ratio, in
    basic CPR, 38–39

Ventilators, nebulizer therapy with, 59
  pressure-cycled, 57
  settings for, 57–59
  time-cycled, 57
  volume-cycled, 57
Ventricular fibrillation (VF), 115–120
  ACLS protocol for, 227
  causes of, 117t
  diagnosis of, 115–117, 117t
  ECG in, *117*
  identification of, 116
  in sudden cardiac death, 7
  mechanical aspects of, 116
  physiology of, 116–117
  prophylaxis of, *18*
  refractory, 119–120
  therapy for, 117–119, *118*
Ventricular flutter, causes of, 121t
  diagnostic criteria for, 121t
  ECG in, *121*
  management of, 120
Ventricular premature contractions (VPC), complex, mortality related to, 8, *9*

Ventricular standstill. See *Asystole.*
Ventricular tachycardia (VT), 121–123
  ACLS protocol for, 228
  causes of, 122t
  diagnosis of, 121–122, 122t
  identification of, 122
Venturi mask, 51
Verapamil, 105
  in ACLS, 216t, 226
  in pediatric patients, 175t
VF. See *Ventricular fibrillation.*
Volume-cycled ventilators, 57
VPC (ventricular premature contractions), complex, mortality related to, 8, *9*
VT. See *Ventricular tachycardia.*

Waveforms, in defibrillation, 74
Witness(es). See *Bystander(s).*

X-ray, chest, post-resuscitation, 209